CONSPIRACY OF H

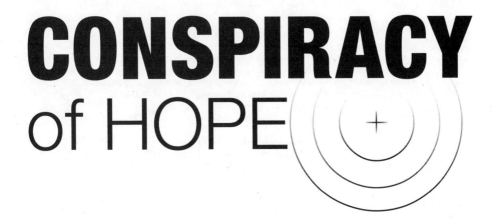

CONSPIRACY
of HOPE

The Truth About Breast Cancer Screening

RENÉE PELLERIN

GOOSE LANE

Edited by Jill Ainsley.
Cover and page design by Julie Scriver.
Cover illustration by Grafissimo, iStock.com.
Printed in Canada.
10 9 8 7 6 5 4 3 2 1

Library and Archives Canada Cataloguing in Publication

Pellerin, Renée, 1949-, author
Conspiracy of hope : the truth about breast cancer
screening / Renée Pellerin.

Includes bibliographical references and index.
Issued in print and electronic formats.
ISBN 978-1-77310-038-8 (softcover).--ISBN 978-1-77310-039-5
(EPUB).--ISBN 978-1-77310-040-1 (Kindle)

1. Breast--Cancer--Diagnosis--Evaluation. 2. Medical screening--Evaluation.
3. Breast--Cancer--Risk factors. 4. Breast--Radiography. I. Title.

RC280.B8P42 2018   616.99'449075   C2018-901268-4
                                                 C2018-901904-2

We acknowledge the generous support of the Government of Canada,
the Canada Council for the Arts, and the Government of New Brunswick.

Goose Lane Editions
500 Beaverbrook Court, Suite 330
Fredericton, New Brunswick
CANADA E3B 5X4
www.gooselane.com

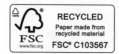

*For the hundreds of thousands of women
who took part in mammography breast screening trials
and to the many dedicated scientists who have devoted
much of their careers to learning the true benefits
and harms of detecting breast cancer early.*

Contents

Introduction   HOW CAN SIZE NOT MATTER?

"What's the use of breast screening?" The question was posed in a deathbed essay that is as poignant and powerful as anything you will ever read in a medical journal. In the context of the era in which Maureen Roberts wrote the piece, it must have been astounding. For ten years, from 1979 until she died in June 1989, Roberts was the clinical director of the Edinburgh Breast Screening Project. But she'd lost faith. "I am in a reflective mood as I lie here in the sunshine at the end of my life," she began, setting the tone for an eloquent plea that the medical community rethink the whole screening idea. The *BMJ* published her article posthumously a few months later.

Based on the knowledge of the day and her own decade of experience, Roberts expressed serious misgivings about the nationwide breast screening program launched in the United Kingdom the year before she died. She acknowledged the studies in the United States and Sweden that were the basis for the UK initiative, research that showed mammography screening reduced deaths from breast cancer by 30 percent. But she urged her readers to also consider other research that did not find benefit. "We all know that mammography is an unsuitable screening test: it is technologically difficult to perform, the pictures are difficult to interpret, it has a high false positive rate, and we don't know how often to carry it out," she wrote. "We can no longer ignore the possibility that screening may not reduce mortality in women of any age, however disappointing that may be." Roberts concluded that the decision to proceed with the program had been premature. "It was clearly a matter of politics, a decision taken in an election year and now out of perspective."

Then she asked, "If screening does little or no good could it possibly be doing any harm? We are all reluctant to face this." One in ten women are asked back for further investigation, she observed. And some 10 to 17 percent of cancers will be diagnosed as non-invasive, something no one knew how to treat. "There is also an air of evangelism, few people questioning what is actually being done," she wrote. "Are we brain-washing ourselves into thinking that we are making a dramatic impact on a serious disease before we brainwash the public?" She worried that women were pressured into being "compliant." "A truthful account of the facts must be made available to the public and the individual patient. It will not be what they want to hear." She went on: "The cur-rently expressed or strongly implied statement that if women attend for screening everything will be all right is not acceptable." Roberts ended on a wistful note: "I feel sad to be writing this; sad because naturally after so many years I am sorry that breast screening may not be of benefit." She was sad, too, for being critical of her valued colleagues, but she said, "They will recognize I am telling the truth."

Maureen Roberts was fifty-three. She died of breast cancer.

The questions she asked have been at the centre of a debate over mammography screening and early detection that has been going on for decades. Does screening really save lives? And if so, at what cost? What are the benefits, and what are the harms? At what age should women begin? Roberts was a physician who was dedicated to screening but who became disillusioned. She was not the first to have doubts, and there have been many more doubters since. The voices most women hear, however, are on the other side of the debate.

Breast screening is a huge industry involving cancer charities, radi-ologists, the manufacturers of imaging equipment, and public breast screening programs. The messaging around early detection is perva-sive. Campaigns in the United States promote giving mammograms for Mother's Day. A hospital in Minnesota holds evening "mingle and mammogram" parties inviting women over forty to enjoy manicures, massages, and snacks along with their breast test. In several countries with public screening programs, women get insistent letters telling them they must go for a mammogram, and if they don't comply, a reminder letter follows. Ontario doctors receive incentive payments depending on how many of their patients go for screening mammograms. Celebrity endorsements help too. Just one example is American singer and breast cancer survivor Sheryl Crow, who teamed up with Hologic, a company that makes 3-D mammography equipment, to promote screening. The message that early detection saves lives has the authority of hefty medical and government organizations behind it. The implication is that women who don't get screened are irresponsible.

Testimonials from breast cancer survivors can also be persuasive. In spite of the messaging, Halya Kuchmij was not a big believer in screening and hadn't had a mammogram in several years. As a documentary filmmaker and journalist, it's part of her job to be aware of current controversies. She was familiar enough with the research to know mammography is not a perfect test, and with no cancer in her family, she didn't think she was particularly at risk. But her doctor had been pressuring her to have a bone density test, a colonoscopy, and mammography. She was sixty when she gave in to her doctor's nagging to get the breast screening done. Six years later, she's adamant it's what saved her life.

Enjoying a mid-afternoon latte and sweet cardamom roll in a small Scandinavian restaurant in west-end Toronto, Kuchmij recalls her reluctance to go for a mammogram. "I didn't bother because there was so much debate about whether they work or not," she confided. "I wasn't convinced that they were helpful." When her doctor's repeated insistence finally made her relent, her attitude about it was casual. She'd just go and get it over with.

Within a few days of her initial mammogram, Kuchmij received a letter requesting that she return for another test. It was careful not to alarm, suggesting that she was being recalled because part of the image wasn't clear and noting that in most cases, nothing is wrong. She wasn't worried at this point. This had happened once before. But when she returned for the second mammogram, it showed something really was there, in the right breast. She was led off to an ultrasound exam and then to an immediate biopsy. Now she was beginning to get nervous. Still, she had no real reason to panic before she got the results, so she went on with her life. She was in shock when her doctor called at five o'clock one afternoon asking that she come to her office right away. Kuchmij didn't have to ask why.

There was something small, just behind the nipple of her right breast. The biopsy had confirmed cancer, and within a week she had an appointment with a surgeon, who explained that he would do a lumpectomy. He was reassuring and so kind that she later felt comfortable asking him to read a little poem to her just before he operated. In spite of the reassurance, she was scared. "Just to hear the C-word," she said, "you imagine yourself in a coffin."

Kuchmij had the surgery on February 27, 2012. According to the pathology report, a mass of suspicious tissue contained just one tiny, invasive tumour, but one lymph node also tested positive, which meant she had a stage-two cancer. The biology of the tumour indicated that it was triple-negative breast cancer, a subtype harder to treat and more likely to spread than hormone receptor–positive (HR-positive) or HER2-positive cancers. HR-positive cancers, the most common, are those fuelled by estrogen (ER-positive), progesterone (PR-positive), or both. They can be treated with drugs that block those hormones. HER2-positive cancers, where the tumours have an excess of a protein that promotes breast cell growth, respond to drugs that inhibit the protein. In triple-negative cancers, the least common, neither hormones nor the HER2 protein is involved, and different treatment is required, typically a combination of drugs delivered intravenously. Kuchmij began her chemotherapy treatments about six weeks after the lumpectomy. After two months of weekly infusions, she had thirty-five rounds of radiation. Her cancer was treated as aggressive.

As she sips her coffee, she casually pats her thick, loosely pinned, dark blonde hair, remembering how strange it was to be bald for six months. "I couldn't even look at myself in the mirror." She had been advised that before having chemo, she should have her hair cut as short as possible to lessen the trauma of losing it. It was still a shock however, and even when she was home alone, she wore a wig or scarf until she got used to having no hair. She's matter-of-fact about it all now, as she lifts the right side of the loose cardigan she is wearing on top of another sweater to show how obvious it is that her breasts are now different sizes. She didn't feel like wearing an insert today. She has considered reconstructive surgery but is in no hurry to do it, being single and not in a relationship. She's working on a film; she is just about to take a short holiday trip with a friend; she seems confident the cancer is behind her. She looks well.

But if it hadn't been for the mammogram, she insists, she wouldn't be sitting here in the restaurant talking about it. During post-surgery follow-up, she had magnetic resonance imaging (MRI), mammography, or ultrasound every six months. An ultrasound technician she chatted with on one such visit told her, "Believe me, if we hadn't found it, you would have been gone in two years, because you had a fast-moving, aggressive cancer." Although none of her doctors made such a definitive proclamation, Kuchmij is certain it's true.

At the time she went for that initial screening mammogram, she already had a symptom of breast cancer but hadn't noticed it. The nipple of her right breast was inverting slightly, turning inward. It was subtle — but obvious once pointed out to her. She simply hadn't been looking. In a way, that, too, reaffirms her belief in the mammogram. It's like insurance against a woman's inability or reluctance to see for herself that something is wrong. Asked for her advice, she would tell any woman to "just go get it." "Because you might find it on your own, but you might not."

Maureen Roberts and Halya Kuchmij represent two different views about breast screening, both grounded in personal experience. They are faces in an irresolvable debate that has as much to do with hope and emotion as it does with science and fact. As a current affairs producer at the Canadian Broadcasting Corporation (CBC), I was aware of the controversy around breast screening. In fact, I had done a television documentary on the pros and cons of mammography in the early 1990s.

There were significant rates of both false positive and false negative results. There was some evidence that screening saved lives, but it was far from definitive. That's when I met Cornelia Baines, who by then had spent a decade as the deputy director of a big Canadian breast screening study and is a central figure in the mammogram debate. But I hadn't realized just how intense and ugly the debate had become until the subject crossed my desk again in 2014. I was leading a team of national health reporters when I learned that a twenty-five-year update of the Canadian study was about to be published in the *BMJ*. (Journalists get advance notice of these things on an embargoed basis.) The article was going to say screening didn't save lives but caused harm by resulting in unnecessary treatment of indolent cancers. I knew it would be a big story. I also knew many find it hard to accept that early detection doesn't work. It's a message completely counter to what we've been taught to believe. Members of my own team found it hard to get their heads around what they were reporting. How could size not matter?

After we aired the story, we received a letter from a scientist complaining that we were wrong to have done so. There was plenty of angry reaction to other media too, including a raft of comments on a front-page article in the *New York Times*. The editor of the *BMJ* also received many letters. In a discussion about these vigorous responses to the study, David Walmsley, then director of news content at the CBC, asked a question that seeded the first thoughts of a book. "Where did the push for mammogram screening begin?" he wondered. Walmsley, currently editor-in-chief at the *Globe and Mail*, has a knack for getting at the *why* of things.

His question nagged at me. Then I learned that Cornelia Baines had received a vicious email from a radiologist. He wrote that he hoped she would be haunted by the faces of all the thousands of women who would die because of her. The nagging in my brain grew into a compulsion to find out the true story about mammograms and why the debate was so heated and nasty. The research took me back to the 1960s and the work of Philip Strax, the radiologist who pioneered mammography screening in New York. His own wife died of breast cancer, and he was determined to end the scourge of this terrible disease. His notion that early detection would solve breast cancer caught on: the American Cancer Society ran with it, and a paradigm was born.

The story of mammography screening is a story about science and medicine. It's a story about hundreds of thousands of women who were participants in screening studies around the world. It's a story about honest differences and sincere efforts to do good. It is also a story about vested interests, money, and greed. When I was working on that TV story in the 1990s, I met a surgeon named Charles Wright who spoke of a "conspiracy of hope." If this sounds extreme, consider that mammography is a multi-billion dollar industry that provides employment to radiologists, creates markets for the latest in imaging equipment built by multinational companies, and perpetuates the bureaucracy and infrastructure of government-run screening programs. Pink ribbon charities that benefit financially from our fear of breast cancer take advantage of paternalistic messaging around early detection. The desire to believe in early detection is intuitive and compelling, with the result that women and their doctors become complicit in the conspiracy, if unwittingly. Charles Wright's language was remarkably prescient.

It's not unusual for scientists to disagree, and controversy in medicine is not surprising. Doctors debate the merits of aggressive blood pressure treatment, the value of statins for cholesterol, whether daily aspirin is good for health, the pros and cons of drinking red wine. After decades of debate, many men and their doctors remain uncertain whether the benefits of prostate-specific antigen (PSA) testing for prostate cancer outweigh the harms. Duelling studies are part of the progression of knowledge. But nothing in medicine has ever generated as much controversy or conflict as mammography screening. The mammogram story is about much more than argument. Sadly, it is often about backstabbing, bullying, and deliberate suppression of information. These are the by-products of fear and hope.

One   TROUBLE FROM THE GET-GO

Cornelia Johanna Baines stood to thank the applauding family and friends who had come to celebrate her eightieth birthday at an elegant dinner in a favourite downtown Toronto restaurant. It was a warm August evening, one of the nicest of that 2015 summer. Inside, where the spirit was equally mellow, the room glowed with admiration. The sixty or so people from a close circle who know her as Corrie were waiting to see what she would say after listening to tributes that were tenderly affectionate and mildly teasing.

Her husband, Andrew Baines, her daughter, Nicole, and son, Nigel, had made toasts to her courage, conviction, energy, and generosity. Her mother was "formidable," Nicole said, listing a string of adjectives describing an invincible, larger-than-life personality: "indomitable" and "opinionated," a person who knows her own mind, happy to convince anyone she is right. A woman of conviction and a champion of causes. Loving and kind. Also neat and efficient: the family calls her "Tidy-up Baines." Much the same was said by the guests at the party who had been invited to submit written comments, cleverly compiled by Nigel in a special booklet he designed as a facsimile of the *Illustrated London News* on the occasion of Queen Victoria's Golden Jubilee. The booklet, titled the *Illustrated Muddy York News, special edition for Cornelia's 80th birthday,* was filled with insightful, moving, and humorous anecdotes paying homage to "Cornelia Regina," a woman strong, determined, wilful, and accomplished.

Her drive to achieve excellence is the dominant theme of the booklet, but her music teacher said it best. Baines earned an ARCT (associate of the Royal Conservatory of Toronto) in piano when she was only seventeen, which any Canadian who has studied formal piano knows is a remarkable feat. When forced to take mandatory retirement from the University of Toronto at age sixty-five, she decided to take lessons again, with the celebrated concert pianist Peter Longworth. Under his mentorship, she tackled one of Beethoven's most difficult works, his Sonata Number 32, in C minor, Opus 111. She sat at her Yamaha baby grand for endless hours determined to perfect it. One day Longworth received a discouraged phone message. "Peter, I am so frustrated. I've been working on this piece now for two years and no matter how much time I spend on it, and how many times I play it, I always make mistakes, and they're always in a different place." Baines had made an important decision. "I'm going to give it one more year, and if I haven't got it by then, I'm giving up." She gave it one more year. "Of course she did get it," Longworth wrote. "We have the recording to prove it."

When Baines rose to respond to all of these respectful comments about her feisty nature, she continued in the same tone. In a playful reference to Shakespeare, she reminded everyone of the challenges that had marked her life. "I suffer not from the slings and arrows of outrageous fortune," she said, "but from the slings and arrows of outraged radiologists." Everyone present knew about some of her outrageous fortune: a catalogue of illnesses from a young age that included chronic kidney disease, lymphoma, and thyroid cancer, among others. They also understood the reference to radiologists. Through most of her career as a medical researcher, she had been at the centre of a fierce debate over mammography screening, all because of her role as deputy director of the Canadian National Breast Screening Study. The questions the study raised about the effectiveness of mammography screening were not ones many in the medical community wanted to hear. To radiologists especially, she was, and continues to be, a targeted enemy. Their slings and arrows have been coming at her for decades.

Controversy has defined most of her academic life, and many have tried to discredit her work over the years. But Baines long ago learned to accept that her role as an adversary was an unavoidable side effect of her research. She is matter-of-fact about having to deal with the critics who dismissed her. She knew the work she and her colleagues did was right, and the critics were wrong. Simple. It's not just that she has a thick skin. Baines is a scientist, compelled to look for truth, and curious. She enjoys the rigours of an honest scientific debate, the search for clues in the data or flaws in the argument, looking for the unanswered questions. She is not one to give in or give up. Her mastery of Beethoven is an apt metaphor for her approach to everything else in life, including her work.

Cornelia Baines is indeed, as her daughter describes, a formidable figure, tall and upright with a stately bearing that belies her age and silvery hair and disguises her chronic health issues. She speaks quietly but with confidence and precision, her speech punctuated by emphatic, long-drawn-out vowels when she's making a point. It was "egreeee-gious," she pronounces, "hil-aaaaarious." She is a well-informed conversationalist with wide interests including music, theatre, and books. She follows politics avidly and applies the same analytical approach to what goes on in the world as she does to science. Her impatience with ignorance and her assertive opinions can be withering to those who don't know her. Those who know her talk about her warmth and sense of humour. A book she wrote about the farm she and her husband bought in Ontario's Grey County in 1970 reveals her more creative side. *Under Sydenham Skies* details their restoration of an old farmhouse, the garden they grew, and the community's indigenous history and colonial settlement. There are stories about the people who became their friends, and favourite recipes accompany tales of country gatherings. Devotion to family threads the narrative.

Baines still goes to work most days, to the University of Toronto office she is allowed to keep as an emeritus professor. Unpaid except for her pension, she is continuing her study of mammography, answering emails from researchers around the world and publishing articles and letters in medical journals. She spends time talking to journalists because she feels it's important to explain the things she knows. In 2013, she took on another controversial issue when she agreed to provide expert opinion on the health effects of wind farms for Ontario's Ministry of the Environment and Climate Change. She testified at several environmental review hearings that no good evidence suggests that wind turbines make people sick. More recently, the Ontario government invited her to serve on a task force on environmental health. She loves this kind of work.

When Baines decided to go into medicine, she could never have imagined she would become a pioneering breast cancer researcher. Her involvement with the Canadian National Breast Screening Study was one of those unexpected life turns with unexpected results. Baines graduated from medical school at the University of Toronto in 1960, at a time when women who wanted to be doctors were considered strange and abnormal, even by, among others, her mother's friends. Cornelia van Erk was an only child who remembers deciding she wanted to be a doctor at age three, partly because she thought that would enable her to assist her parents in providing her with a brother or sister. Also, her grandmother suffered from a condition known as "milk leg," a colloquial term for a blockage of veins in the leg called thrombophlebitis. As a child, she helped to dress the ulcers this caused.

A fascination with all things medical grew. Her library book choices taught her about scientists such as Marie Curie, Louis Pasteur, and Frederick Banting, and reading about exotic diseases such as leprosy captivated her. At age fourteen, she got a summer job in the pathology department of the Banting Institute at the University of Toronto, where she observed the dissection of specimens. She remembers vividly a huge breast plopped onto the cutting board and kidneys being sliced. The following year she worked in the pathology lab at Toronto Western Hospital, feeling very grown-up in a white coat. Before she entered medical school, she got a job in another lab at the Banting Institute and met Charles Best, the co-discoverer of insulin. This proved a less interesting experience: she spent a lot of time feeding rats, mushing up a mixture of dog food and grains with her bare hands while huge white rabbits stared at her. A few years later, another job involving unpleasant experiments that caused injury to rats put an end to any interest in further lab research.

Accepted into medical school in 1953, when there was a quota on women and Jews, she excelled. She was at the top of her first pre-med class. But when she graduated, a kidney condition called glomerulonephritis meant she did not have the physical stamina required to do a rigorous internship. Instead, she went to work as a cancer research fellow at Toronto Western Hospital and later as a teaching assistant at the University of Toronto. She had married her classmate Andrew Baines and had her first child when they were both still studying to be doctors. In the mid-1960s, the young family went first to the United States and then to France so that Andrew could pursue doctoral studies. Back in Canada after three years abroad and now the mother of a second child, Baines became a consultant at the *Medical Post*, a national news magazine for physicians. Then around 1970, she met the chief of medicine for Toronto Western Hospital. He wanted her to work in his outpatient department and persuaded her to do an internship at his hospital. Internships were less physically daunting than ten years earlier, and she was finally able to practise medicine.

Being in the outpatient department was a revelation. She was not impressed by how some of the doctors worked. For instance, she came back after being away to find one of her patients had been put on antihypertensives, medication for high blood pressure. She believed from her work at the *Medical Post* and from continuing medical education programs that, as she puts it, "You never put someone on an antihypertensive the first time you saw them." She had learned it was best to take several blood pressure readings during repeated appointments to get a more accurate assessment because some people have white coat syndrome, meaning that their blood pressure goes up just because they are in the doctor's office. "And here were people taking my patients and putting them on antihypertensives, and I didn't think that was very good practice," she says, with a sigh of incredulity.

At about the same time, she remembers, the hospital was going through an accreditation process, and increasingly she could see the importance of quality-control procedures, auditing, and observation of care. She enrolled in the groundbreaking and internationally renowned Design, Measurement and Evaluation program at McMaster University in Hamilton, Ontario, a program founded in 1968 by a young David Sackett, a physician and scientist who is considered the father of evidence-based medicine. Baines obtained a master's degree in epidemiology, the science that studies patterns of disease and risk factors and evaluates health policy aimed at disease prevention. At McMaster, she learned the value of meticulous methodology, the importance of recognizing bias in research, and respect for evidence. She had intended to return to Toronto Western Hospital after earning her master's degree in 1980 but instead went to Oxford, England, with her husband, now a University of Toronto professor on sabbatical. There she found a position in epidemiology. A year later, preparing to return home, she wrote to the University of Toronto to inquire about work in her new field. That's when she got the attention of Anthony B. Miller and learned for the first time about a Canadian breast screening study. It was 1981.

Miller is the epidemiologist who made the Canadian National Breast Screening Study happen. On the third floor of the McMurrich Building, a typical ivy-covered, early twentieth-century building on the University of Toronto campus, he was leading a team already at work for eighteen months. The McMurrich Building is nestled among the structures that hug Queen's Park Crescent, on the west side of the Ontario Legislature. It was originally the anatomy building, completed in 1923. A tree-lined path meanders elegantly to an arched entrance with big wooden doors, giving the building a sense of legacy and purpose. But when Cornelia Baines walked up that path on a summer day for a meeting with Anthony Miller, barely knowing anything about the Canadian breast screening study, she wasn't thinking about any kind of legacy. She was just looking for work.

As a young doctor in England, Miller had treated women with advanced breast cancer and was involved in researching a drug that might stop the progression of the disease. "It was terribly sad because we didn't really have an impact," he reflects. He was upset over his inability to help the women, but they were so nice to him it was as if they were helping him cope with their disease. The experience inspired in him the desire to investigate the causes of breast cancer, leading him to a research path. He abandoned clinical practice to become a scientist.

After nine years at the British Medical Research Council, where he learned the intricacies of conducting clinical trials, Miller transplanted his career to Toronto. In 1971, he accepted a position as assistant executive director at the National Cancer Institute of Canada, where he also became director of a clinical trials group and an epidemiology unit. In those days, Toronto was a staid and conservative city with a small-town feel, not much noticed internationally. Nevertheless, it was a good opportunity. One of the things that attracted Miller to Canada was the existence of cancer registries. The cancer registry in Saskatchewan, dating back to the 1930s, was one of the earliest in the world, and it has one of the longest-running databases on cancer anywhere. Other provinces had followed Saskatchewan's example. The registries were established to collect the data needed to justify expensive radiotherapy treatments in cancer centres. Such data, says Miller, are a gold mine for epidemiologists. When you've got these data, he explains, you can assess differences — for example, the differences between age groups. Before Miller came to Canada, the International Union Against Cancer had collaborated with the International Agency for Research on Cancer to publish a book called *Cancer Incidence in Five Continents*. Many subsequent volumes of this book have updated the data over the years, but Miller still has volume one in his library, and in it are data from five different Canadian cancer registries.

Miller's arrival in Toronto coincided with another gold mine for cancer research. In his State of the Union address in January 1971, President Richard Nixon declared the American "War on Cancer." He promised to seek an appropriation of an extra $100 million for a campaign to find a cure. "The time has come in America when the same kind of concentrated effort that split the atom and took a man to the moon should be turned toward conquering this dread disease," the president famously proclaimed. At the end of that year, on December 23, he signed the National Cancer Act. More Americans die of cancer each year than had died in all of World War II, Nixon said before he applied his signature to the document. The legislation ensured plentiful amounts of new money for research. Some of that money would go toward mammography screening in the United States, and, inevitably, trends in American medical practice rubbed off on Canada. Anthony Miller was in the right place at the right time.

Miller is in his mid-eighties now, but it's easy to imagine a young physician who cared profoundly about the women with breast cancer he couldn't save. To his friends, close associates, and family, he is known as Tony. His handshake is warm, his smile friendly, and his voice soft. He is slender and fit, a man who still travels the world for work with the World Health Organization and to meetings about cancer. In his eighty-third year, he logged trips to England, Ireland, Egypt, Iraq, Qatar, Saudi Arabia, France, Germany, and Colombia. He is properly English still, with an educated accent. At home, he is casual but elegant in a navy cardigan, stylish blue plaid shirt, beige slacks, and expensive-looking caramel-coloured shoes. He is surrounded by mahogany furniture and Persian carpets. A grandfather clock chimes on the quarter-hour.

At the National Cancer Institute of Canada, Miller was one of the country's medical authorities. Soon after his arrival, he was invited to take part in a national committee of radiologists looking at the possibility of introducing breast screening to Canada. Although it recognized mammography as a good tool to aid in diagnosis when a clinical exam found something suspicious in a woman's breast, the committee felt more research was needed before instituting screening programs for healthy women and recommended to the then Department of National Health and Welfare and to the National Cancer Institute of Canada that they should support a study. A follow-up committee in Ontario agreed that a study should be done. All Miller needed to do now was find the money.

Miller travelled around the country speaking to the heads of cancer centres and to radiologists in various urban centres that might participate. He organized three pilot studies with funding from the National Cancer Institute of Canada. One of those was about recruiting. The first thought was to get family physicians to recruit women into the study, but Miller and his team weren't sure that would work. So he asked some volunteers, among them his wife Sheena, to use the telephone and personally invite people to go for screening at Women's College

Hospital in Toronto, explaining what they were trying to do. Sheena Miller delights in saying she got an extremely positive response from the women she called. Previous involvement with politics in England had taught her the art of persuasion. It was fun. This little pilot study taught them that they should apply the personal touch and reach out to women directly. They needed tens of thousands to volunteer, so finding the right recruitment approach was key.

There had been only one previous study on mammography screening. The Health Insurance Plan of Greater New York (HIP) study, done in the 1960s, involved sixty thousand women between the ages of forty and sixty-four. Half were invited to receive four mammograms and clinical breast exams annually, whereas the other half, the controls, were left on their own to do whatever they would normally do. The trial investigators reported a reduction in mortality of 30 percent among the women screened compared to those not screened. But here's something important in understanding the mammography debate: the benefit was not seen in women aged forty to forty-nine. Mammography did not appear to be saving lives in those women under fifty. What could explain this result? The researchers and their observers decided there were simply not enough women in that age group in the study to produce conclusive findings. Because so few women in their forties die of breast cancer, it would take a very large number of participants to show any real differences between the study group and the controls.

There was another issue with the HIP study. The women in the screened group were given both a clinical breast exam and a mammogram, but when the results were tabulated, the researchers could not say whether mortality reduction was due to mammography, the clinical breast exams, or both. What extra benefit did mammography offer?

The study Anthony Miller designed needed to answer two critical questions. First: will screening women under age fifty save lives? The Canadian researchers estimated that they needed fifty thousand women in that age group to resolve the lingering issue from the New York research, which seemed to indicate that screening was not effective in younger women. Second: in women over fifty, does mammography confer benefit over and above a clinical breast exam? The researchers estimated they needed forty thousand women aged fifty to fifty-nine to answer that question. Ninety thousand women would have to be cajoled into taking part. A trial of this size, huge by any standard, was unheard of in Canada. It was a massive and ambitious proposition.

Women would be involved in the study for four years. The women aged forty to forty-nine would be randomized into two groups: the study group would have four annual mammograms plus clinical breast exams following the initial screen; the control group would be given clinical breast exams and then assigned to normal community care and not invited to screening. The women aged fifty to fifty-nine would be randomized into either a study group that received clinical breast exams plus mammography once a year for four years or a control group that would receive the clinical exams only.

In 1979, Miller obtained funding to begin his study the following year, but in just two screening centres, one in Quebec City and one in Toronto. The study ran into trouble before it began. Never mind the obvious challenge of recruiting so many women. Never mind the challenge of raising the money. A new hurdle suddenly appeared. In the fall, just months before the study was to start, Miller accepted an invitation to Roswell Park Memorial Institute in Buffalo, New York, to give a talk about diet and breast cancer. While there, he took the opportunity to mention his study on breast screening, intending only to describe briefly what it was about. When a statistician named Irwin Bross got up, Miller expected to be attacked for his notions about diet. But to his surprise, Bross attacked him for poisoning women with radiation.

Bross was the head of the Roswell Park Memorial Institute's biostatistics department and a public health advocate. He believed the ionizing radiation from mammograms was dangerous, and he predicted that mammography would result in an epidemic of breast cancer in young women. When he learned about Miller's study, Bross wrote to the *Globe and Mail* and the CBC to let Canadians know the National Cancer Institute of Canada was making what he called a "terrible mistake." The *Globe and Mail* printed Bross's comments, and CBC Radio's *As It*

Happens aired a debate between Bross and Miller. The *Ottawa Citizen* joined the skirmish with a scare story headlined "100,000 Guinea Pigs Sought for Cancer Fight." The story's opening paragraph read: "In an effort to control the breast cancer epidemic in Canada the National Cancer Institute is looking for 100,000 guinea pigs to take their chances with the ill effects of radiation." For Miller and the screening study, it was a public relations nightmare.

Many scientists considered Bross extreme in his view, on the fringe in arguments about radiation hazard. In an unusual note appended to an article Bross and his colleagues wrote for the *American Journal of Public Health*, the editor admitted: "Dr. Bross stands virtually alone in defense of his data and the interpretations he places on them." Bross would not agree to a peer review of the article, so the journal also published a critique from another expert. Nevertheless, he made himself heard in the Toronto media, and his arguments alarmed the Toronto Board of Health. The board called Miller to a hearing to justify the risk he was inviting women to take and to explain what precautions would be in place. "If it is possible that even one woman may die of radiation induced breast cancer as a result of a mammogram from this study, the study is unethical," one board member stated. Miller was fighting a brush fire that threatened to engulf his entire research plan, just one month before he was going to start his study in Toronto. He sought advice from a US expert, summoned support from radiation physicists in Toronto, and managed to satisfy the Board of Health that the risk of breast cancer from mammography radiation was low. But the bogeyman was unleashed, and Miller feared that the women he needed for the study, and their doctors, would need some extra persuasion. That's when Cornelia Baines entered the scene.

The study went ahead in Quebec City and Toronto in January 1980, as planned. The next year, with additional funds, three more centres opened in Montreal, Hamilton, and Winnipeg. Recruitment was slow, taking twice as long as expected. When Baines became deputy director in August 1981, the study had already been under way for more than a year and a half, but its future was uncertain. Baines remembers that when she sat down with Miller before he hired her, he warned that the study could likely be over by the end of the year. He recalls the moment a little differently. "I might have made an off-the-cuff remark, which could have been, 'You know if we don't succeed, we've got another four months to show this,' because I think that was when I had to go for more money." Regardless, together they were confronting a huge challenge. The study needed to operate in fifteen centres. They were far from that goal, and the additional money they needed would be difficult to raise if they couldn't demonstrate success in the existing centres. Recruitment quickly became Cornelia Baines's first priority, not only because she needed to secure her job. She believed the reasons for the study were important. They had every expectation that early detection of breast cancer would save women from death. All they had to do was prove it.

Baines needed to figure out what was stopping women from coming into the study, and she sought to identify the barriers to recruitment. One was the family physician. From personnel in the breast screening centres, she collected anecdotes of things said by doctors. Some physicians feared that the screening centres would diminish the demand for their own services. "When I received the letter which told me my patient had had a normal screening examination I was hurt and angry. It seemed to me my patient was expressing lack of confidence in my examining skill," one doctor reportedly said. "I don't want any other surgeon recommending to me that certain diagnostic procedures be performed on one of my patients, it's unethical," said another. A third said: "I disapprove of submitting normal women to mammography." And finally: "I wouldn't let my wife go in the study." Baines also received reports of women who dropped out of the study because their doctors asked them to.

Clearly, the study needed buy-in from family doctors. Baines and Miller published an article in *Canadian Family Physician* in March 1982 explaining what the study was about, the goals and the protocols, and why it deserved support. In the same issue of the journal, Miller wrote an editorial appealing to doctors to support the study and encourage their patients to take part. It was a sincere request for help.

As predicted, the radiation fears persisted, particularly in Toronto, where active campaigns attempted to shut the study down. Torontonians of a certain age will remember Morton "Morty" Shulman. Shulman was Ontario's chief coroner in the 1960s and later served as a member of the Ontario Legislature after writing a book about how to make money in the stock market. As a politician, he was outspoken, opinionated, and usually digging up dirt. He was an irascible figure with a certain kind of love him/hate him charisma. In the late 1970s, he hosted his own television show, *The Shulman File*, where he further branded his persona with controversial and argumentative interviews, and had a column in the *Toronto Sun* newspaper. Morty Shulman didn't like the breast-screening study and talked about radiation frequently on his program. Cornelia Baines was convinced that he was determined to get the study terminated. Another opponent who got media attention was Sister Rosalie Bertell, a Grey Nun from Buffalo, New York, who was an award-winning environmental activist and considered an expert on ionizing radiation. Because her mother was Canadian and she lived so close to Canada, Bertell was a Toronto media favourite. Cornelia Baines was listening to local CBC Radio one day and jolted in stunned surprise when she heard Bertell say having a mammogram would age a woman by one year. It was a distortion of risk statistics and nonsense but, says Baines, "devastatingly effective."

Radiation phobia was part of the culture. In March 1979, the United States had experienced its worst nuclear accident in history, at the Three Mile Island nuclear plant in Pennsylvania. The accident caused a partial meltdown. It took days to get the reactor under control, and it took months to figure out exactly what had happened. Hysteria was the natural public reaction. Amazingly, the Three Mile Island accident happened just twelve days after the release of *The China Syndrome*, a movie about a fictional nuclear breakdown starring Jane Fonda, Michael Douglas, and Jack Lemmon. The fear of mammography wasn't out of place in the context of the time. And if Bertell, the anti-nuclear nun, spoke out against mammography, it would have some impact on the study.

Baines fought back. She felt that the best defence against the critics was to be articulate, accurate, and very well informed. She happily spent time answering questions from reporters. She's always felt that as long as they have questions, she should answer them. She remembers the day she got her chance to answer questions from the inflammatory TV doctor Morton Shulman. It was an important interview. "He probably thought I was going to be shivering in my boots," Baines recalls. "So he made his introductory statement, and I looked at him and said, 'Dr. Shulman, everything that you have said is totally wrong.' I was then able to go forth and say what I wanted to rather than answer a question that was stupid and unanswerable."

Media appearances were one element of her recruitment strategy. Baines also did a lot of speaking to women's groups, doctors' groups, and anyone who would invite her, playing the role of the study's ambassador. She assembled a panel of high-profile patrons who agreed to support the screening trial publicly. The panel included the wife of Ontario premier Bill Davis, former Ontario lieutenant-governor Pauline McGibbon, highly acclaimed writer June Callwood, and Celia Franca, the artistic director of the National Ballet of Canada. The Canadian Cancer Society helped with publicity. There were media ads and public-service announcements. The study team sent out thousands of personalized letters to women in Toronto and followed up with phone calls to appeal to potential volunteers directly. In 1982, the study received a great boost from Canada's minister of national health and welfare, Monique Bégin. She signed up with the centre in Montreal to become a participant in the study and made it possible for the study to send out a nationwide recruitment appeal as an insert included with monthly family allowance cheques. Bégin's support also made it easier for Miller to get centres set up in Alberta and British Columbia.

The pamphlets urging women to join in had an optimistic and persuasive tone, signalling the high hopes for mammography screening. "Get informed, be examined," the leaflets exhorted. "You'll be helping to save the lives of thousands of women everywhere. Not to mention, perhaps, your own," promised one. "Breast cancer is the number one killer of women in their 40s and 50s. This we know. We also know that the earlier breast cancer can be detected, the greater the chance for cure. We know that mammography can reveal abnormalities up to four years sooner than they can be felt. And we know that mammography can detect cancers so small that extensive surgery may not be required." The literature also made it clear that researchers had yet to answer the question "Can screening by mammography reduce death from breast cancer in women forty and over?" That was why women should step up. Those who agreed to participate were promised attentive care for five years. And in recognition for her contribution, every woman in the study received a "Lease on Life" certificate, acknowledging that "She has not only unselfishly helped to further a Study that it is hoped will help increase both life expectation and quality of life, for women who develop breast cancer.... But herself will have acquired knowledge and experience that may help give her too a longer, healthier lease on life." Cornelia Baines and Anthony Miller signed each certificate, by hand, in red ink. It helped to relieve some of the tedium of departmental meetings.

The recruitment strategies got results. Miller was able to secure the funding needed for ten more study centres in 1983, making fifteen in all, in Nova Scotia, Quebec, Manitoba, Ontario, Alberta, and British Columbia. The task of recruiting ninety thousand women, enough women to fill a huge arena such as Wembley Stadium in London or the Cotton Bowl in Dallas, was completed in March 1985. The sheer size of the effort was impressive. So was the cost. Miller obtained $20 million for the study — a formidable sum by Canadian research standards at a time when research grants rarely surpassed a few hundred thousand dollars. "That was unprecedented," he says now, "but I can tell you it wasn't easy."

A small medallion, still pinned to the wall of Baines's university office some thirty years later, is a reminder of that hectic, exciting time when she was the de facto emissary for the study. It hangs from a pink ribbon, about ten centimetres long, positioned at eye level among an array of family photos and academic memorabilia. It's a "professional commitment award" from the Canadian Breast Cancer Foundation, given to her in 1988. Back then, the foundation was a fledgling charity, only two years old, dedicated to raising money for breast cancer awareness campaigns and research. It was also a time when enthusiasm for provincial breast screening programs was growing. In March 1988, Miller and Baines participated in a high-powered workshop asked to consider the evidence for screening on behalf of provincial ministers of health. The workshop recommended province-wide screening programs in dedicated centres for women aged fifty to sixty-nine, where they would be offered mammograms and physical breast exams every two years. British Columbia became the first province to initiate a breast cancer screening program, which it did that very year.

Meanwhile, the results of the Canadian breast screening trial were eagerly anticipated as much was at stake for those wanting to launch mass public screening programs. The buzz would soon turn negative. Miller and Baines had faced almost insurmountable hurdles to get the study under way, but their success in addressing the early controversy around radiation from mammography and overcoming the difficulty in recruiting such a large number of women did not mean the end of their problems. Bigger trouble lay ahead. It would be a while before they had enough data from the trial to publish any results, but Miller and Baines saw something puzzling and alarming almost from the start.

When they began their research, they both fully expected that mammography would show the desired result, that because it detected cancers before they could be felt, treatment could begin earlier and lives would be saved. To any rational person, that would seem intuitively logical. But as they began to track the data, they noticed something that didn't make sense. In the part of the study involving women aged forty to forty-nine, what was happening was completely the opposite of what they thought they would see. More women in the screened group, the mammography group, were dying of breast cancer than in the unscreened group. How could that be? At this point, the numbers of deaths were very, very small, and there was no way to know whether the trend would continue. It might be an anomaly, a fluke. But it was worrisome.

The study's advisory panel included Richard Margolese, a prominent oncologist and surgeon from Montreal; Sam Shapiro, an American statistician who had also worked on the earlier New York study; and other experts who advised the National Cancer Institute of Canada and the Department of National Health and Welfare. The advisory group could have stopped the study but concluded that, given the small mortality numbers thus far, it was best to continue. Baines thought the excess mortality was bizarre — she called it the "mortality paradox" — and it bothered her enormously. But it seemed to her that screening, not the trial, was doing harm. "If you had asked me then I would have said well, it's a good thing we are doing the trial because it's revealing things that we otherwise wouldn't know." She explains that "when you begin a trial, you have prior evidence that indicates what your trial is trying to answer is compelling enough that you can ethically continue with the trial."

The early mortality results became hugely controversial. In April 1991, Anthony Miller discussed preliminary findings at the Second International Cambridge Conference on Breast Cancer Screening. He provided figures on the excess deaths, comfortable that he was in a private meeting. But someone leaked the figures to the press. Two months later, London's *Sunday Times* ran a front-page story with a sensational headline: "Breast Scans Boost Risk of Cancer Deaths." To suggest that there was cause and effect, that mammography was the cause of the deaths, was completely wrong because the researchers were still trying to figure out how the excess deaths could be explained. But the error persisted and generated further comment. Then an anonymous editorial in the *Lancet* picked up on the *Sunday Times* piece and created even more consternation about the excess deaths. Miller and Baines were on the defensive before their research was ever published.

Meanwhile, they had become involved in a dispute with a high-profile radiologist at Harvard University, Daniel Kopans. When Miller developed the protocol for his study, he consulted widely with radiologists in Canada and the United States; some continued as advisers and would have known about the puzzling mortality paradox. He also did what no other breast-screening researcher did before, or has done since, and instituted an external quality review of the study's mammograms. Miller invited Kopans to take part, and in 1990, Kopans was one of the authors of a paper reporting the results of that review in the *American Journal of Roentgenology*, an influential radiology journal. The review outlined some technical problems and the measures taken to correct them. But to Miller's surprise, Kopans took the unusual step of independently writing a commentary, published in the same edition of the journal, describing the mammography in the study as poor quality. Kopans had turned on him. He was attacking the study's credibility. Kopans has persisted in dismissing the Canadian mammograms and the Canadian study ever since, and to this day, he continues to fire off a note of criticism any time the Canadians report anything from their study.

When Anthony Miller and Cornelia Baines finally published the initial results of their work in the *Canadian Medical Association Journal* in 1992, they had already been under siege. It got worse. Their report, a seven-year follow-up on the ninety thousand women in their study, concluded that mammography screening did not reduce deaths from breast cancer, neither in the group aged forty to forty-nine nor in the group aged fifty to fifty-nine. Not finding any benefit in the younger women was consistent with what other research had shown. But finding that mammography conferred no more benefit than clinical breast exams in the older group was unexpected even though these were still early results and things could change in time.

The reaction in Canada was explosive. Breast screening programs women could access without referral from their doctors were now in place in two Canadian provinces. The Canadian Breast Cancer Foundation was heavily promoting screening. Trust in early detection was becoming culturally engrained. It was unthinkable to radiologists, to physicians, and to women that finding a tumour before you could feel it wouldn't make any difference. They didn't believe it. They couldn't believe it. Media reaction was equally negative, with headlines such as "Despite Breast Cancer Study, Save Your Life and Get Tested," "Mammograms Useful Despite Study Results, MD," and "Doctors Defend Breast X-rays." Experts quoted in those stories repeated the badmouthing Miller and Baines were hearing from Daniel Kopans. Quebec radiologists declared that there were serious flaws in the study. Doctors in British Columbia complained that the technology was old.

Critics who were angry at the message vilified the messengers. Cornelia Baines was stunned by vituperative phone calls from people telling her she should commit suicide because she was doing so much harm. "I never, ever imagined that whatever results we got when we published them would not be respected, accepted, and treated civilly. Especially by people we had interacted with over the years of the study. It never entered my head."

The medallion dangling from the pink ribbon pinned to her wall has served as a reminder of those interactions, a reminder of a more innocent and hopeful time before the mammography debate got ugly. Cornelia Baines and the Canadian Breast Cancer Foundation would soon part ways, and become bitter foes. By the time they first published in 1992, Miller and Baines were already facing influential and powerful opponents. They would continue their research. They would keep following the women in the study and report again.

But the real mammogram wars had only just begun.

Two   PAP TEST FOR THE BREAST

"This patient has a breast cancer, and that's what breast cancer looks like on mammography." Derek Muradali is demonstrating how radiologists read mammograms. "In this case it looks like a big lump, like a nodule," he explains as the cursor settles on the screen. His visitor squints at the screen, unable to discern the lump in what looks like a fuzzy white cloud. Muradali patiently continues with other examples. If you want to see what mammography looks like, he's an excellent person to ask. As the radiologist-in-chief for Cancer Care Ontario's breast screening program and the head of the Division of Breast Imaging at the University of Toronto, Muradali is one of the most expert radiologists there is. He's been reading mammograms for nearly twenty-five years.

His office at St. Michael's Hospital is clearly not a place where he spends a lot of time. The desk is bare, and nothing is on the walls. Normally, he would be in the radiology department, examining newly completed mammograms. The images he's putting up on the screen now are ones he's selected for instructional purposes, when he gives talks. They're culled from his own experience and represent real patients, without any of the usual labelling that would identify them. He hopes it's not too chilly; it's a bitter November day, and he's had to turn on the heat. Dressed in a casual, short-sleeved polo shirt, he jokes that he might shiver through the interview.

The dark areas are the fat in the breast, he says, focusing on the screen. The white areas are the glandular tissue and the milk ducts. He looks for vague masses or bright little flecks of calcium in the white areas. "Most calciums in the breast are benign, and in fact all women have some calcium in their breasts. But when cancer occurs in the breast, the calcifications change." When a woman gets screened, the radiologist looks at two images of each breast. If something suspicious shows up, she's called back for additional, more targeted images obtained by compressing the breast more than in the initial screening tests, making a suspicious area easier to see. If the concern persists, a diagnostic ultrasound is ordered. Muradali pulls up two images to demonstrate the contrast between a mammogram finding and the same finding with ultrasound. The mammogram shows a little white dot. The ultrasound confirms more clearly that there is a mass. Ultrasound cannot image the entire breast, but it's useful in checking selective small areas, and its sound waves can distinguish between a solid mass and a benign cyst filled with liquid.

Next he brings up three mammograms that illustrate how subtle the images can be. "They kind of look the same, right? These little nodules there, there, and there?" One little nodule is a cyst, essentially a harmless little bag of water. The nodule on the second mammogram is a cyst that bled into itself, also harmless. The nodule on the third is breast cancer. The differences are impossible to see with an untrained eye. "That's why mammography is so hard and breast imaging so difficult," Muradali says. "Mammography is a very good tool, but it's not a perfect test. It really isn't. We will miss breast cancers on mammography because it can be very difficult to interpret. And it's because of cases like this. The whole of breast imaging is a very complex, very difficult field." He compares mammography to computed tomography (CT or CAT). "A CAT scan of the abdomen, it's pretty obvious. If there's a cancer, boom, you find it. In mammography there are lots of shadows, lots of things overlap, the tumours are often very small. Sometimes you just won't see it."

The challenges of reading images of the breast may explain why mammography was a relative latecomer to the field of radiology, decades after x-rays were first discovered. The German physicist Wilhelm Roentgen happened upon the x-ray accidentally in 1895. He was experimenting with an electron discharge tube and a fluorescent screen when he was surprised to see that he could create an image of the bones in his hand on a piece of photographic film. The experiment created electromagnetic radiation, resulting in mysterious rays that penetrated his flesh to illuminate his hand's skeleton. He did not know what the rays were — hence "x-rays." Also known as the Roentgen ray, Roentgen's discovery quickly became an important medical tool for examining broken bones. Roentgen, credited with creating a medical miracle, earned the first Nobel Prize in Physics in 1901. In 1913, a German surgeon created the first x-ray images of female breasts, experimenting with samples extracted from mastectomies. Other researchers in Europe and South America then experimented with actual patients but could not find a technique that worked well on soft tissue. The pictures were not good enough, and breast imaging did not catch on.

In 1930, an American radiologist created a flurry of renewed interest. At Strong Memorial Hospital in Rochester, New York, Stafford Warren was investigating chest x-rays when he found he could get an image of the breast by moving back a few feet. He came up with a new technique that involved having women lie on their sides and raise their arms to have a breast x-ray and published the first US study to recognize it as a tool in diagnosing breast cancer. The flurry of initial interest faded when other radiologists did not have the same success in locating tumours. The quality and consistency of the images were still in question, and neither radiologists nor surgeons were ready to endorse this uncertain technology with unpredictable results.

One researcher persisted. Radiologist Jacob Gershon-Cohen in Philadelphia toiled away at using x-rays in breast cancer diagnosis and refining the technique. He stressed the importance of compressing the breast to get a clearer image. As early as 1937, he advocated the use of x-rays not just for diagnosis but also to screen asymptomatic women. In 1956, he began a five-year screening program at Philadelphia's Albert Einstein Medical Center, in which thirteen hundred women underwent a screening x-ray every six months. It was the most extensive such program in the United States up to that time. Gershon-Cohen is often cited as the father of mammography, even though his method was not widely adopted because, just as with the earlier Warren technique, other radiologists had difficulty replicating it and achieving images of comparable quality.

In the 1950s, a French researcher developed a prototype for a dedicated mammography unit with a device that compressed the breast to obtain better pictures. Research in Uruguay contributed to the technique's refinement. Still, it was rarely used in the United States. Robert Egan, at M.D. Anderson Hospital in Houston, Texas, began to look into mammography in 1955, and, not convinced that the technique used by others was providing accurate enough images, he developed his own. In 1960, he published the results of a study, and others who reviewed his work found his images sharper and more detailed than Gershon-Cohen's. More importantly, the Egan technique was easier for other radiologists to learn and duplicate, and it soon became the standard as interest in mammography revived. Another factor was that in contrast to Gershon-Cohen, who received no government funds for research, Egan managed to win institutional support. In 1963, the US Cancer Control Program partnered with the National Cancer Institute (NCI) and M.D. Anderson Hospital to conduct a nationwide study of the Egan technique to verify its clinical applications. In 1965, the results of that study reinforced the reliability of the method and established that other radiologists could, with five days of training, replicate Egan's work. The US surgeon general applied his handwritten signature to a short preface endorsing the published findings, signalling that finally, half a century after a German surgeon produced the first grainy, fuzzy images of breast tissue, mammography's acceptance in medicine was assured.

With that stamp of approval from the surgeon general, the American College of Radiology got in line to add its endorsement of diagnostic mammography and proceeded to establish a basic training program for its members. These two important endorsements, however, did not include the use of mammography for screening. In fact, the authors of the study concluded that the application of mammography in screening would need to be evaluated by further research. All the women involved had palpable lesions and were already scheduled for biopsy; therefore, the study wasn't a test of early detection. Yet Gershon-Cohen's earlier work had shown that mammography could find cancers no one could feel. It was inevitable that the radiology community's acceptance of diagnostic mammography would lead to a greater enthusiasm for screening. But would finding the cancer early make a difference? The question was still unanswered, and, ultimately, if the point of early detection was to save lives, researchers needed evidence that mammography would indeed do that. It was possible that screening would only ensure that women with cancer would live longer with the knowledge of it. It's what scientists call lead time.

Philip Strax was a mammography pioneer who understood the need to test the assumptions about early detection. Strax was a general physician who learned radiology so that he could apply it in his New York practice in the 1940s. A tragedy in his own family was the turning point that not only set the direction for his own career but also led to the widespread adoption of mammography screening in the United States.

The life of Philip Strax is one of those quintessential American stories in which greatness arises from humble beginnings. Born on January 1, 1909, Strax grew up in Brooklyn, where his father, an immigrant from eastern Europe, worked in the garment industry sewing suit pockets. The family was poor. The eldest of five children, Strax loved to recount the time when he slept on two chairs in the kitchen because the family was so crowded in their tiny three-room apartment. His Jewish parents fostered learning and hoped that at least one of their children would become a doctor. Remarkably, three of them did, with Philip being the first, followed by another son and a daughter. An exceptionally bright student, Philip finished high school at age fifteen, and one of his teachers helped him earn four scholarships to attend New York University, prophesizing in a letter that this unusually talented young man might someday succeed in conquering "the dreaded scourge of cancer." After getting a bachelor's degree, Strax financed medical school working as a photographer and part-time newspaper reporter. He graduated at the age of twenty-two and after a general internship opened a private practice and married Bertha Goldberg. It was 1933, in the middle of the Great Depression, and in that first year of practice, Strax earned just six hundred dollars. The only way to manage was to live with Bertha's parents, which the couple did for at least two years, even after the birth of their first child. As Strax built up his practice, he thought he should learn to do x-rays to better help his patients. He took a postgraduate course in radiology and installed an x-ray machine in his office. Later he would become head of radiology at City Hospital as well as professor at Mount Sinai School of Medicine.

In 1947, Bertha died of breast cancer at age thirty-nine, a mother with four small children. Ruth, the eldest child, was only seven, but she remembers that her mother passed away after a short illness, perhaps within six months. She also remembers that, in an era when it was thought best not to talk about death around children, her father presented a stoic countenance. Pictures of Bertha disappeared from sight, and within a year, Strax remarried, and normal family life resumed. But inwardly, his loss affected him deeply. At the time, the plague that was breast cancer killed half of its victims within five years, and he felt he needed to do something to spare his two young daughters from their mother's fate. Saving women from breast cancer became his life's mission. At age seventy-nine, long after he might have retired, he was still practising medicine in Florida, examining women at a breast cancer detection centre he set up in the city of Lauderhill. A writer for the Palm Beach newspaper *Sun Sentinel* visited him for a feature story in 1988, the year he won a prestigious Kettering Prize for cancer research. He told her the breast was a marvellous and complicated creation. "If only the goddamn thing wouldn't get into trouble," he said. "I'm going to find out what causes that trouble. Then I'm going to quit." By all accounts, Philip Strax was a driven, dedicated, and deeply caring physician, a tireless crusader with a gentle, reassuring voice. His son Richard describes his father as a humanitarian who repeatedly told his children they must leave the world a better place. For Strax, success was never about money or prestige. It was about saving women's lives.

Not long after his wife's death, Strax learned about Robert Egan's work with mammography. As head of a radiology department, he thought he should find out more and took his family on a car trip to Houston to visit Egan personally. Strax was amazed when Egan showed him x-rays of breasts that had cancer, cancer a woman could not feel yet was visible on film. That's when the idea sparked in his mind that maybe there was a way of finding breast cancer early, and maybe that would make a difference. He became convinced that he could save lives and began inviting women — "gals," he called them — to come to his office to get screened. He set up two clinics in New York where women could get mammograms for free. Richard Strax remembers that when he was nine or ten years old, sitting at the dining room table in their Long Island suburban home doing school work, his Dad was there too, studying stacks of breast x-rays.

Surgeons of the day generally resisted mammography, more comfortable with their own skills at palpating breasts than with a technology they didn't trust. But Strax was a convert. He wanted to develop screening programs. He also understood the need to prove that screening would indeed have an impact on those dreadful mortality numbers. He decided to do a proper study. He convinced a statistician from the health insurance industry and a breast surgeon to join him in an endeavour that would turn out to be a milestone. Sam Shapiro was the director of research and statistics for the Health Insurance Plan of Greater New York. Louis Venet was a surgeon at New York Medical College. They found an ally in Michael Shimkin, the director of field studies at the NCI, who had also been thinking a study was needed to determine whether screening had value. The NCI agreed to fund a screening trial.

That trial began in December 1963, and over the next two-and-a-half years, Strax, Shapiro, and Venet enrolled sixty thousand women aged forty to sixty-four from the membership of the Health Insurance Plan of Greater New York. The study became known as the HIP study. The women were randomized into two groups: half were assigned to the study group and received a mammogram and clinical breast exam annually for three years, whereas the other half, the controls, were assigned to usual care. The researchers estimated that they would need to follow these women for five to ten years to determine whether screening saved lives. In hindsight, the project was bold, visionary, and breathtaking. The HIP study was the first randomized trial of screening mammography in the world and the only one of its kind that would ever be conducted in the United States.

Strax, Shapiro, and Venet reported preliminary findings in 1966 in *JAMA: The Journal of the American Medical Association*, indicating that, so far, they had found twenty-three confirmed cancers in the study group and fourteen in the control group. Among the cancers in the study group, they reported that sixteen, or 70 percent, of the twenty-three cancers had not spread to involve any lymph nodes. Of the fourteen cases in the control group, eight, or 57 percent, had no lymph node involvement. It seemed that screening was capturing the cancers earlier; it was promising news. Five years later, they were able to analyze mortality statistics. In March 1971, the study team reported in *JAMA* thirty-one deaths from breast cancer in the screened group compared to fifty-two deaths from breast cancer in the control group. There were twenty-one fewer deaths in the screened group. It was even more promising news.

Later it would be said that in the HIP study, screening reduced the numbers of deaths from breast cancer by 40 percent. The researchers themselves did not use that 40 percent number in their 1971 report, but it represents an interpretation that became common in the medical literature. Forty percent refers to what is called the *relative* difference between fifty-two and thirty-one. There were twenty-one fewer deaths; twenty-one is 40 percent of fifty-two. The relative difference, however, exaggerates the findings. Another way to look at these kinds of numbers is to consider the *absolute* difference. In absolute terms, there were thirty-one deaths out of 32,000 (0.09 percent) in the screened group compared to fifty-two deaths out of 32,000 in the control group (0.16 percent). Look at it that way, and you see the difference is small, only 0.07 percent. Even very small differences, however, can matter in diseases that are as common in the population as breast cancer. You can see why advocates for screening would prefer the more impressive-looking relative number.

Strax, Shapiro, and Venet exercised restraint. They did not exaggerate. Although their results were encouraging, they wrote, "it must be emphasized that the observations are preliminary, and more time, possibly ten years of follow-up, is needed to establish whether the effect of the screening program is short-term or long-term." The numbers were too small, over too short a period of time, to provide any hard conclusions. And there was something more: the differences in deaths occurred only in women over age fifty. The New York team ended its 1971 article on a note of "cautious optimism," suggesting that it would be prudent to accelerate advances in technology and training in anticipation of "the broad demand for periodic breast examinations that might emerge within a few years."

Scientists around the world were watching the progress of the HIP study with keen interest. Canadian epidemiologist Anthony Miller was in the audience at a meeting in Italy of the International Union Against Cancer when Sam Shapiro presented some of the research from the study. Miller had an issue with the way Shapiro was analyzing his data; Shapiro wanted to talk. It marked the beginning of an important professional relationship. Shapiro invited Miller to come to New York to look at the data, and Miller ended up travelling there every six months or so to help with some of the analysis, in particular to help analyze the deaths to determine if the women who died really died of breast cancer and not some other cause. Miller was impressed: "That team was dedicated," he recalls. He got to know them well, and they became friends. Miller would later consult these New York friends when he designed his own study in Canada.

Arthur Holleb also had a keen interest in the HIP study. In 1971, Holleb was senior vice-president for medical affairs and research at the American Cancer Society. A cancer surgeon, he had come to the cancer society in 1948 to help promote screening for cervical cancer using the Pap test. From the Pap test campaigns, researchers learned many lessons about funding training programs, clinical trials, routine screening in hospitals, and patient education programs. The Pap test was credited with dramatically reducing mortality from cervical cancer, and the American Cancer Society was credited with changing attitudes in both the medical community and the public. By campaigning directly to women, it created a demand for the test. It also created a profile for itself. The American Cancer Society had a cause.

The success of the Pap test made Holleb a fervent believer in cancer screening, and he saw an opportunity to promote widespread screening mammography in the same way. In the fall of 1971, he issued a press release titled "Toward Better Control of Breast Cancer" to announce plans to mount a breast-screening demonstration project. "No longer can we ask the people of this country to tolerate a loss of life from breast cancer each year equal to the loss of life in the past ten years in Viet Nam. The time has come for greater national effort," he declared. "I firmly believe that time is now." Holleb's idea was to invite women for free breast screening at different centres to demonstrate the technology and make women and doctors aware that mammograms could detect breast cancer. His planning was well timed. Two months later, Nixon signed the National Cancer Act into law, which gave the NCI generous funding for cancer control programs.

Three forces at play in the mammography story converged that year. The HIP study issued promising findings from a randomized trial, the National Cancer Act resulted in a lot of new money for programs, and the American Cancer Society's experience with the Pap test primed it to launch a major breast screening program. On February 5, 1972, the American Cancer Society voted to support, for two years, twelve breast cancer detection centres at a variety of hospitals, universities, and community institutions. That initial plan soon changed. Knowing that the NCI now had money for just this kind of thing, Arthur Holleb went to see Nathaniel Berlin, one of the institute's directors, and they made a deal. The NCI would contribute $6 million annually toward funding twenty-seven breast cancer detection centres for five years. The goal was to recruit 270,000 women ages thirty-five to seventy-four. The Breast Cancer Detection Demonstration Project was ready to go in 1973.

Suddenly, the world's most influential cancer research body, the NCI, a federal government organization, was aggressively selling to the public a technology that just one randomized trial in New York had tested. The only study done up to then had failed to prove that early detection had any impact on mortality among women under fifty. Yet the Breast Cancer Detection Demonstration Project was inviting women as young as thirty-five to mammography screening. The HIP study researchers had also cautioned that, notwithstanding promising results in women over fifty, they needed more time to see whether screening would have long-term results. The science was not there, at least not yet. The demonstration project barrelled ahead regardless.

With the infusion of resources from the federal government, a whole new medical industry was about to take off. Radiologists would be trained. Clinics would be established inside and outside the demonstration project, and demand for screening would grow. The makers of imaging equipment were encouraged to develop even better mammography technology, and they promoted it. In an ad in a medical journal, Kodak put forward "a hopeful message from industry on a sober topic." Picker X-ray touted its latest machine: "Mammorex II can see it before she can feel it."

As the demonstration project got under way, Philip Strax presented an update to his study at an annual meeting of radiologists. Again, he reported no difference in mortality between the screened group and the control group in women under fifty. Among the women over fifty, there were sixty-three deaths in the control group and forty in the study group. He concluded that mammography reduced mortality by one third in the older women. Years later, the NCI's Nathaniel Berlin said he didn't care that the HIP study had no effect on breast cancer deaths in women under fifty. The numbers didn't bother him, he told an interviewer for the institute's own oral history project. The interviewer also pointed out that the demonstration project was not set up as a research project with a control group and would not advance any knowledge about the impact of screening on mortality. Berlin didn't care about that either. The leaders of the demonstration project simply believed that the HIP study had already confirmed the merits of mammography.

Regardless of the results for younger women in his study, Philip Strax remained committed to the philosophy of early detection. In a much more personal, kindly, physician-like tone, he published a hundred-page book called *Early Detection: Breast Cancer Is Curable* in 1974. It was a book for women, with a powerful message: women who did not take control of their own health by getting screened were just like the typical absent-minded professor who walked into traffic without looking and got killed. "Every woman carries within her body a built-in hazard — the risk of breast cancer," Strax wrote. "She may ignore that risk, like our unfortunate professor, and become a victim of it, with disastrous results to herself and her family. Or she may be constantly on her guard, aware that she may be affected, but with assurance that early detection may save her life. Which course should you follow?" Women, he wrote, are tempted to sweep their anxieties under the rug. He described his book as a clarion call to women to abandon such a fatalistic and passive attitude. "The long stalemate in reducing mortality due to breast cancer has been broken by new and painless techniques of detection. How effectively these techniques are used depends on women themselves," he insisted. "It is up to every woman to cooperate actively in assuring her own survival."

The paternalism of the time is obvious. Not so obvious is the role this little book must have played in getting women to participate in the demonstration project. Strax was part of that project, leading one of the twenty-seven centres involved, at the Guttman Institute breast detection clinic he established in 1968. In his book, he acknowledges with gratitude the inspiration and help given him by Arthur Holleb and Nathaniel Berlin, "whose foresight is helping to prevent needless deaths of women from breast cancer." He donated his share of sales revenue to the American Cancer Society. Holleb was equally effusive in a note on the back cover: "This book is a long overdue testimonial to the value of modern technology in the earlier diagnosis of minimal breast cancer.... This book should be required reading for every woman — it is not only educational, but it may also save the reader's precious life."

The relationship between Philip Strax, the NCI, and the American Cancer Society was a cozy collaboration. The demonstration project successfully got women into the mammography centres. In 1974, in the program's second year, it received a tremendous public relations boost when both Betty Ford, the first lady, and Happy Rockefeller, the wife of the vice-president, within two weeks of each other, went public with the news that they had just had mastectomies. They joined in the chorus urging women to take care of themselves and get screened. Their courageous disclosures made talking about breast cancer and mastectomies, once taboo, acceptable, and the awareness they raised had immediate impact. The "Betty Ford blip" encouraged so many women to have themselves checked that the incidence of breast cancer went up by 15 percent.

But although the publicity generated a lot of enthusiasm for mammography screening, things would not go smoothly for long. One person at the NCI had a lot of questions about the Breast Cancer Detection Demonstration Project. John C. Bailar was the deputy associate director for cancer control, a role he took on as the institute was implementing the National Cancer Act of 1971. "When I got there this whole breast cancer demonstration project was dropped on my desk, and they said do it," he recalled. But no one would answer his questions. "It wasn't that I got answers I didn't like, I didn't get any answers at all." After a few months, he sent a long memo to the then director of the institute listing approximately three pages of concerns. He received no response. It was frustrating to be supposedly in charge when he couldn't get anyone to talk to him. "I think their idea was the program was set in stone, and my job was to write cheques. It wasn't the way I looked at things."

Bailar had concerns about the harms mammogram radiation might cause, particularly to the younger women in the project, and about what the project had done to minimize those harms. He wondered why the effects from radiation hadn't been investigated more actively. He also had questions about the results of the HIP study, about the lack of impact on mortality in younger women, and about the fact that it was not clear in the older women what benefit mammography had beyond the clinical breast exam, which was also being done. And how could there be any research value in a demonstration project that didn't have a control group? Bailar was a physician and a cancer researcher, a highly respected epidemiologist who had spent many years assessing cancer statistics. He began to think there was more to the demonstration project than simply a concern about reducing breast cancer. "I recall very vaguely hearing one or two comments about how this was such a marvellous fundraising device," he said. "That really set me thinking about it." An American Cancer Society slogan asked the public to "Fight cancer with a check, and a check book." Bailar noted that when the society campaigned for donations, it used the demonstration project as an example of the public good it was doing.

John Bailar was a lone voice — at first. After he began to speak out against mammography, he noticed that he was excluded from official discussions. Yet he persisted. When the media got hold of a paper he'd submitted to the *Annals of Internal Medicine,* his criticisms resulted in a big story and a public outcry. The NCI would eventually come under so much fire that some administrators started to wonder what they had gotten into when they agreed to support the demonstration project. The NCI announced that routine screening of women under fifty would stop. Then it commissioned reviews of both the HIP study and the demonstration project and in 1977 called all parties together for a consensus conference. That conference set the course for mammography for the next decade and prepared the groundwork for the Canadian National Breast Screening Study that Anthony Miller launched in 1980.

The evangelical rhetoric that screening saves lives had momentum and would grow louder in spite of the lack of evidence that it was true. It would never go away. But John Bailar had inspired an important conversation.

Three   THE MAMMOGRAM WARS BEGIN

Standing before the elite of medical minds in America, not intimidated by the importance of the moment and ready to challenge their assumptions, John Bailar knew exactly what he wanted to say. It was September 14, 1977. The National Institutes of Health (NIH) had decided that it was time to make some decisions about breast screening and had invited leading cancer experts and clinicians to review the science and come to Bethesda, Maryland, to share their opinions. Bailar had long been waiting for this day. After all, if it hadn't been for him, this powerful gathering might never have happened. He had been questioning the Breast Cancer Detection Demonstration Project since the file had landed on his desk five years earlier when he was acting director of the cancer control program at the NCI. As his concerns with the project grew, he dared to make them public. He had pestered his superiors to listen to those concerns and do something about them. Now, at this consensus development meeting on breast cancer screening, he had the audience he wanted.

A large man carrying some extra paunchy weight on his six-foot-two frame, he was a formidable figure at the podium. He wore glasses, had bushy brown hair and a thick moustache, and recalled that he was probably dressed in a white shirt with a jacket and a necktie "from years before." He was forty-six years old. As he reflected on that day nearly four decades later, his voice was clear, assured, and forthright, and his speech was simple and direct. The transcripts of the meeting indicate that he spoke plainly then too. He stood before some five hundred people in the main theatre of the sprawling NIH campus, on the main floor of Building 10, the world's largest clinical research hospital. The red Chinese fabric covering the walls of the recently redecorated Masur Auditorium cast an elegant glow on the proceedings. Although Bailar described it as a solemn occasion, he remembered that he had a fairly easy attitude at the podium after many years of teaching and presenting papers at meetings, and he "was having a pretty good time, since there can be joy in needling the stuffy."

The NIH had never held a meeting like this before. In the foreword to the published transcript, NIH director Donald Fredrickson called the meeting an experiment in a new way to come to decisions about scientific matters that had wide social implications. The old way was the tried and true but slow way of one study building on the evidence of another, of one clinical trial pointing to the direction for the next, until there was what Fredrickson called "doctrinal wisdom." The rapid pace of technological development called for quicker decision making. The doctrinal wisdom around breast screening had not yet been developed, but it had become popular, and questions about cost, safety, and effectiveness needed timely answers. What was the benefit of screening? What was the risk?

The three-day consensus development meeting brought together everybody who was anybody in the breast cancer community in the United States. The Canadian cancer researcher Anthony Miller was there too. Their task was to assemble the latest data and suggest breast screening policies based on the current state of knowledge. Sixteen medical, legal, and ethical research leaders, four women and twelve men, were appointed to a panel to hear evidence from a wide spectrum of experts that included radiologists, representatives from the American Cancer Society and the Breast Cancer Detection Demonstration Project, epidemiologists, oncologists, surgeons, and breast cancer patients. The event was open to the public.

Rose Kushner was an invited expert who, like John Bailar, was not afraid to be cast in the role of rebel. She would not have come to this meeting with strong views about screening, but she defiantly advocated for women to be informed about their choices and involved in decisions about their health care. She was the new voice of breast cancer, a woman who dared to question whether her doctor knew best. Three years earlier, when she was forty-five, Kushner discovered a small bulge in her breast while having a bath. Skilled as a journalist and medical writer, she dove into researching breast cancer. She was appalled to learn about the surgery and how it usually went. The surgeon would put the woman under, remove some of the tumour, and have it analyzed immediately while she was in the operating room. A pathologist would do what's called a frozen-section procedure, where the tissue sample is put in a cryostat machine to cool it so that it can be sliced, stained, and examined under a microscope within minutes. If it was cancer, the surgeon would do a mastectomy right then and there, and the woman would not know what happened until she woke up. It was known as the one-step mastectomy. Most often, the standard practice was the brutal radical mastectomy adopted in the early 1900s, involving the removal of chest wall muscle and underarm lymph nodes. It's what Betty Ford had in 1974, just months after Kushner faced her own diagnosis of cancer.

Kushner insisted on a different plan. She wanted to have a biopsy first and then, if it was cancer, a modified, more conservative mastectomy that she'd learned some surgeons were beginning to do. She made eighteen telephone calls before she found a doctor who would agree to remove just the lump. Later, with a confirmed diagnosis, she did have a mastectomy. But she was infuriated by a patronizing system where a doctor would make a decision on a woman's behalf, and she began a determined campaign advocating for a two-step approach with less radical surgery and for women to have more control of their treatment. She wrote a book about the experience, and wanting to help other women, she established the Breast Cancer Advisory Center, which they could call or write to for information. She continued her research and became an authority on breast cancer diagnosis and treatment. Kushner is credited as the person most responsible for putting an end to the one-step mastectomy, and she arrived at the consensus conference as a famous cancer survivor with the kind of notoriety that comes with being an agent for change. She was interested in radiation issues and

appointed three experts to examine specific issues: one to review the benefits reported in the HIP study, the second to look at the radiation risks of mammography, and the third to re-examine the pathology of the breast tumours in the HIP study.

A series of cascading events in 1976 would ultimately lead to the consensus development meeting and Bailar's opportunity at the podium. His paper, "Mammography: A Contrary View," finally appeared in the *Annals* in January. "I regretfully conclude that there seems to be a possibility that the routine use of mammography in screening asymptomatic women may eventually take almost as many lives as it saves," he wrote. "Screening by medical history and physical examination also will probably provide much or most of the same benefit without risk from irradiation, at least in women under some fairly high age limit."

The American Cancer Society, facing questions from journalists at its annual meeting in March, admitted that women in the demonstration project had not been told of any radiation risks. On July 1, the NCI took administrative control over the demonstration project, and two weeks later, the first of the NCI's three committees delivered a draft report. The institute promptly assembled a meeting to discuss it and invited journalists and the public. That committee, led by Lester Breslow, dean of the School of Public Health at the University of California, Los Angeles, reviewed the HIP study and looked at the possible harms of radiation. Breslow boldly recommended that screening of women under fifty should stop. He also recommended further clinical trials to ascertain more precisely what benefit screening offered. On the subject of radiation, he recommended standards for mammography that would ensure the least possible radiation required to get images of sufficient quality to detect tumours. Directors from the breast-screening demonstration project balked, and *New York Times* writer Jane Brody captured the tone of the meeting in a story the next day headlined "Mammography Test for Cancer in Women Under 50 Defended." Nevertheless, on August 23, the NCI and the American Cancer Society jointly issued interim guidelines to the twenty-seven breast screening centres involved in the demonstration project, asking them not to screen a woman under age fifty unless she and her physician felt it was necessary. The project had promoted screening for all women starting at age thirty-five. The new guidelines signalled a fundamental change in direction.

On September 23, 1976, the *New England Journal of Medicine* upped the temperature of the controversy when it published an investigative report from health journalist Daniel Greenberg. Through a freedom-of-information request, Greenberg dug up internal memos and briefing documents showing that others at the NCI besides John Bailar had been unhappy about the demonstration project from its beginning. They just hadn't been public about it. In a meeting summary, Philip Strax was reported to have said, "Mammography was of virtually no value in women under fifty years of age." The institute had received letters from cancer experts who said the demonstration project's inclusion of women under fifty was wrong and "close to unethical" and the project was ill-conceived. Greenberg discovered in another meeting summary that Nathaniel Berlin had said that both the American Cancer Society and the NCI would gain a great deal of favourable publicity because they were bringing research findings to the public and applying them, and that would assist in obtaining sorely needed funds for basic and clinical research. It was exactly what John Bailar had been worrying about: a possible ulterior motive for the demonstration project that had nothing to do with saving women's lives. Then in November, Sidney Wolfe, head of the Health Research Group in Ralph Nader's influential Washington consumer lobby, Public Citizen, exposed the damning information that the demonstration project's mammography equipment was producing wildly different levels of radiation. Wolfe had learned that a third of the machines exposed women to unacceptable doses.

These revelations fuelled a debate in the media, in medical journal editorials, and in letters to the federal health department and the NIH. Those who had enthusiastically marched ahead, espousing the creed that a woman who avoided screening was risking her life, were now being held to account. The NCI and the directors of the demonstration project held ongoing discussions about controlling levels of radiation and providing women with information about risks and proper consent forms. Early in 1977, the NCI set up a fourth committee, chaired by Mayo Clinic surgeon Oliver Beahrs, specifically to review data from the demonstration project. He was to investigate whether there was anything that should be added to the information available from the HIP study.

Meanwhile, the interim guidelines meant to halt the screening of women under fifty didn't seem to have much effect, at least not immediately. In April 1977, the project centres reported their screening rates. Seventy-five percent of women between thirty-five and forty-nine in the project returned for an annual screening despite the decision to no longer screen women in this age category. The guidelines said "for women of high risk because of family history, reproductive history, prior breast cancer, et cetera, the benefits as well as the risks of x-ray mammography should be fully explained to the woman and the final decision be made between her and the physician." The problem was that the definition of *high risk* was open to interpretation. Arthur Holleb, the leading proponent of screening at the American Cancer Society, said the women at high risk were those who had chronic cystic disease of the breast, lumps or thickenings, nipple discharges or abnormalities, personal breast cancer histories or past diagnostic breast surgery, family breast cancer histories, early menstrual histories, no pregnancies or a first full-term pregnancy at age thirty or older, and women with an unusual dread of breast cancer, or cancer phobia. How cancer phobia was linked to the risk of getting cancer was unclear, but screening advocates argued that mammography was important to reassure women who did not have cancer.

According to Holleb, about 80 percent of women between thirty-five and fifty fell into these "high-risk" categories, and he thought they should have at least one baseline mammogram. Adopting such a wide interpretation of risk meant essentially ignoring the guidance to halt screening of younger women. At the time, the lifetime risk of breast cancer was thought to be 7 percent. Critics thought the idea that 80 percent of those young women were at high risk was patently ridiculous.

John Bailar told the consensus meeting it was mathematically absurd. "We simply cannot have everybody, or even a majority, at risks that are significantly above average," he said. But, apparently, Holleb's message had kept women coming into the screening clinics. In mid-1977, the NCI revised the guidelines to make the definition of *high risk* more narrow and specific. Only then did the number of women screened in their forties go down.

So there he stood: John Bailar, the scientist with the pesky questions that others didn't want to ask, challenging the captains of the war on cancer. Sitting before him in the Masur Auditorium on that day in September 1977 were Philip Strax and Sam Shapiro; Benjamin Byrd, chair of the American Cancer Society; Richard Lester from the American College of Radiology; the sixteen members of the consensus development panel; and several hundred radiologists, clinicians, and researchers with strong views on the benefits or the harms of early detection. Bailar's words were blunt: "I am concerned by the fact that radiation required by mammography will eventually cause many deaths from breast cancer, the very disease we want to detect and treat." Then he added, "I am even more concerned about the exceedingly optimistic expectations of what mammography can accomplish. Mammographers themselves seem to be among the worst offenders in this regard. Many simply do not have a realistic view of their procedures' limitations. My interest in this entire problem was stimulated first not because the risks were being ignored but because the public was being misinformed about the benefits."

Bailar had looked closely at the HIP study's results. The women in that study had clinical breast exams along with their mammograms. What difference did mammography make beyond a simple clinical exam? The research hadn't answered that question. "Would a screening program without mammography be successful?" he asked. "It has been said that many women participate in the BCDDP [the demonstration project] only because of the attraction of the extensive, newly developed machinery. If so, if what you could call the pizzazz of the mammographic equipment itself is so important in attracting screenees, something is fundamentally wrong with the way the program has been promoted to the public."

Bailar went on to parse the numbers in the HIP study. It found 299 cancers in the screened group and concluded that thirty-eight more women survived than would have normally survived without screening. Other observers had concluded that of that thirty-eight, mammography contributed to survival in no more than one third. No more than 4 percent of the 299 women with cancer might have survived because of mammography. Then, Bailar said, roll in other factors, such as lead-time bias or the possibility of finding indolent cancers that would not develop, and no more than 2 or 3 percent of cancer cases could be said to benefit from mammography. And if one considered the radiation risks over a lifetime, women under fifty with a low risk of cancer should not be screened, he said. Bailar carefully enumerated a list of problems and then suggested that the answers to those problems were already apparent in the study's data from 1972, well before the American Cancer Society mounted a major effort to promote mammography screening. "The most careful disinterested observers have generally concluded that the benefits of mammographic screening for breast cancer are limited," he argued, "and the risks must be given much weight."

Bailar spoke about *minimal cancers*, a term he said was often used but one he objected to. "While it is sometimes used to refer to small but clearly genuine cancers, it has more often included lesions that are either entirely benign or of dubious malignant potential," he noted. "I believe that such lesions should be clearly and honestly labelled. When their significance is undetermined, that should be stated. To call them 'minimal cancers' is to confuse doctors, mislead the public, and, again, overstate the value of screening." After methodically outlining all the issues troubling him about screening healthy women, he made a final plea that well-considered recommendations to stop screening women under fifty not be outweighed by emotional appeals from well-meaning and concerned physicians.

Several directors of the screening clinics addressed the room in exactly the way John Bailar foresaw. Their appeals were indeed emotional. It was clear that these were men with a commitment to an idea, sincere in their fervour, their gut instincts overruling science. Myron Moskowitz was the head of the screening centre in Cincinnati, one of the earliest involved in the demonstration project. When he got his chance to present statistics from his own centre showing how mammography could pick up minimal cancers far earlier than a physical exam, he made an impassioned plea: "For the first time in the history of medicine, we have been able to detect with reasonable regularity internal malignant neoplasms while they are still at the microscopic level. To discard this advance out of hand because of presumed risk, in my opinion, would be imprudent." He said the core issue was whether there is a stage of breast cancer that is curable that can be found on a mammogram. He was convinced that mammography's ability to find those cancers and change the course of the disease was unequivocal, and he argued that women should be aggressively screened beginning at age forty. Indeed, he was right about the core issue, whether finding a cancer early made it curable. That was the whole point of the three-day discussion. But Moskowitz was disregarding the fact that there was no evidence that screening women in their forties saved lives. He was a believer, even though the only data available, data from the HIP study, didn't support his belief.

Myron Moskowitz doesn't remember very much about that meeting now, but the early days in his screening clinic are vivid. The chaos he describes is a reminder of how experimental the whole field was at the time the demonstration project was launched. When he heard that the American Cancer Society was planning to open mammography centres, he put together a consortium of three different hospitals in Cincinnati, secured funding, and got the clinic up and running. "That was August '73. Some dates you remember like your birthday," he says emphatically. As a radiologist, he had used mammography for diagnosis, not for screening. It was a difficult technique that required processing film images by hand. As the demonstration project got under way, a new type of mammography unit that delivered lower radiation doses and was easier to use became available. Moskowitz recalls that demand for those units increased quickly, but as it often is with new equipment, there were glitches, and the screening clinic was so busy there wasn't time to wait for technical support or new parts. They improvised. He describes the unit as having a long cone at the end of which hung a balloon that compressed the breast. "If you couldn't find balloons, or the balloons burst, you could get condoms and blow them up. That's what we wound up doing often."

He chuckles when he thinks about how ill-prepared they were for the volume of mammography they were suddenly doing. They might have done one or two a week in an average practice before the screening program began. Now the clinic was expected to do forty a day. "It was a side show," he says. Not many people were trained to do the x-rays or read them, and in order to do forty a day, they had to run clinics at nights and on weekends. Moskowitz remembers long delays when equipment broke down. "There was always some damn thing and the women were sitting there waiting and waiting and waiting." The tasks of efficiently reading a mass of mammograms, getting reports out to people, collecting the data, and calling women who needed to be notified of abnormalities were unrehearsed. It took a while to get things moving smoothly. Moskowitz also remembers that it was easy to get women to come to the centre because the American Cancer Society publicized it well and there was a lot of interest, especially after Betty Ford and Happy Rockefeller went public about their mastectomies. A local patron donated a truck and a van to operate a mobile clinic in a poorer part of Cincinnati, and Moskowitz recalls that middle-class women, who normally "wouldn't be caught dead in that neighbourhood," called in for appointments when they couldn't get into the main centre.

But at the consensus meeting in 1977, the sixteen-member panel heard that women were no longer so enthusiastic, and the project centres were losing them. The controversy over the risks and benefits of mammography had frightened and disturbed women all across the United States. Philip Strax, the kindly mammographer who pioneered screening, ignored the results of his own HIP study and spoke to the panel with words of eloquent desperation. At the Guttman Institute in New York, part of the operation was engaged in the demonstration project, but a substantial part was his own separate clinic. Many of the sixty thousand women who had been in the HIP study continued to get mammograms, for free, at that clinic. Strax estimated that suddenly, in the previous year, ten thousand women did not keep their appointments. He guessed that there were now twenty-five Guttman Institute casualties, twenty-five women with undetected breast cancer because of hysteria over radiation. "The damage to women both emotionally and potentially physically in future missed early cancers may already be considerable. If we destroy the value of mammography in the eyes of women, we will be guilty of permitting 25 percent or more of breast cancers to progress with the potential loss of a golden opportunity to save the lives of a substantial number of women." He pressed the members of the panel: "Women both young and old with their male companions look to you through their source of medical information, the media, for guidance in the most serious problem they face, breast cancer....I hope your deliberations will make it possible for you to say to the women: you are faced with a serious problem. At least part of the solution is available. Early detection of breast cancer leads to much improved survival and possible cure. If you are forty years old or older be sure to get yourself a regular complete examination which includes mammography....I strongly urge you to get the average woman off the hook now." Belief in an idea trumped the results of his own screening trial.

After hearing some stunning information put forward by the committee analyzing data from the demonstration project, Rose Kushner had an emotional appeal of her own to make. The analysis included a pathology review of 506 lesions classified as minimal, lesions smaller than one centimetre. The review determined that sixty-six of those lesions were completely benign and twenty-two were borderline. Kushner was enraged to hear that most of the sixty-six women with benign lesions had had mastectomies, half of them radical mastectomies. "I am sure they are very grateful that they owe their lives to the mammographs," Kushner said, "and these lucky women no longer have to worry about recurrences and metastasis. I hope somebody is going to tell them they didn't have cancer after all and it was just a terrible mistake." She said radiation concerns paled into insignificance "in light of these unnecessary amputations and lousy pathology." It wasn't an attack on screening or even the breast screening demonstration project, but she did, as John Bailar had, ask the meeting to consider the complications and implications of treating women aggressively for minimal cancer. Women, she said, had to have better reasons to trust their doctors.

In 1977, some surgeons were promoting breast-conserving surgery along with radiation or chemotherapy, but these now-routine adjuvant therapies were new and experimental. The state of the art was evolving. There were also unanswered questions about the natural course of the disease. For instance, how long did it take for a cancer to take hold and grow? Was there a latency period where even the x-ray could not see the tumour? Could the cancer have already spread even though it could not be detected? And were all the tiny tumours seen on x-ray lethal ones? We still don't have all the answers. But in the 1970s, debate about appropriate treatment was going on at the same time as debate about early detection. It was incredibly complicated. For the radiologists who spoke at the conference, the value of early detection was without question. For others, such as John Bailar, the only real measure of value was whether or not it saved lives. And if some of the "minimal cancers" the screening proponents were so proud of finding might not be ones that anyone needed to worry about, women were being treated unnecessarily. Without naming it, he was talking about overdiagnosis, when mammograms find cancers that might otherwise never be noticed, never grow, and never cause a problem. Bailar's argument about minimal cancers was remarkably prescient. Overdiagnosis is one result of early detection that today is much better understood.

But the consensus meeting had a job to do. The NIH wanted to formulate a clear policy that would end the hysteria and confusion the demonstration project had created and give women and doctors guidance about what was best going forward. The four committees the NCI set up all reported to the meeting that there was no evidence that screening women under age fifty saved lives. But there had only been one study. Many presentations to the panel suggested that more research was needed: a bigger trial than the HIP study that could be more definitive about the benefits of screening women under fifty and a trial that could measure whether mammography truly offered greater benefit than regular physical exams.

In the end, the panel concluded that the evidence to justify screening women under fifty in the demonstration project was insufficient. It said the evidence regarding women over fifty rested on the combination of physical exam and mammography, and no evidence indicated to what extent either a physical exam or mammography alone contributed to a reduction in mortality. The panel acknowledged improvements in radiology technique and a reduction in radiation doses and agreed that the risk attributable to radiation was lower among older women, but the data were inconclusive about what dose, exactly, was safe. The panel made no recommendation about how to proceed with future clinical trials but "deplored the lack of clear-cut data on the efficacy and the risk-benefit ratio of screening for women under fifty years of age" and said clinical trials would be important to resolve outstanding questions.

In the following years, the NIH would go on to hold consensus conferences routinely on a wide number of subjects, from HIV/AIDS to prostate cancer to diabetes, conferences that would set national guidelines for medical practice. But this first attempt to develop scientific consensus was historic, not just because it was trying to come to grips in an innovative way with a current sticky issue but also because it established a path to follow for future complicated issues.

The Breast Cancer Detection Demonstration Project was funded for five years, and as was planned, it ended. But the early-detection paradigm was set, and the growth of breast screening was inexorable. Private clinics made mammography screening an important part of their practice and flourished. Philip Strax continued to operate the Guttman Institute clinic in New York and went on to operate another mammography screening clinic in Florida. Myron Moskowitz had joined the demonstration project fully aware that the findings of the HIP study had shown no benefit in young women and that there were questions the study did not answer. But he also thought, *It's obvious it's going to go on; we might as well be part of it.* When the project ended, he maintained a private screening clinic in Cincinnati and became influential in the promotion of mammography as a radiology specialty. Today, he reflects that the demonstration project may not have been the best idea, that it should have been a real research project, another big randomized trial. "It would have bypassed a lot of the arguments that we wound up with," he says. But he's never given up on the idea of early detection. "There is one thing very clear from this whole brouhaha," he wrote in an email. "If we can lower the stage of detection we can add time to life. Now we have to find the most efficient way to do that."

Myron Moskowitz would become part of the Canadian story when Anthony Miller invited him to take part in a qualitative review of the mammograms in his national breast-screening study. Its purpose was to answer the very questions posed by the consensus panel, and Miller and Moskowitz talked about expanding it into the United States. That never happened. Despite the calls for further research in the United States, the will to make it happen did not exist. The NIH declined to fund another project.

John Bailar was relieved that the consensus conference in 1977 had come down to "almost 100 percent" of where he hoped it would be. He left the NCI in 1980 to join the faculty at the Harvard School of Public Health, where he was also a statistical consultant for the *New England Journal of Medicine*. He then spent several years as the chair of epidemiology and biostatistics at McGill University in Montreal before going to the University of Chicago in 1996 to become chair of its new Department of Health Studies. While he was at McGill, he became the centre of another controversy when he authored an article in the *New England Journal of Medicine* declaring Nixon's War on Cancer a failure. In 1997, he made headlines once more with another paper in the same journal, one he co-authored with a medical student, titled

"Cancer Undefeated." In it, they denounced "blind faith" in screening and argued for strategies aimed at prevention to replace early detection.

Bailar died of cancer in 2016, at the age of eighty-three. He was a highly respected, brilliant statistician and epidemiologist who promoted evidence-based medicine his whole career. The debate on mammography screening is only part of his legacy. But he began it. And it fell to Canadian researchers Anthony Miller and Cornelia Baines to pick up where he left off, to do what he asked at the conference, to do the research needed to answer his questions.

Rose Kushner continued to be an untiring activist. She wrote several books, became an advocate for lumpectomy as an alternative to mastectomy, championed legislation that would ensure that the US Medicare system paid for screening mammograms, and for six years served on the National Cancer Advisory Board, appointed by President Jimmy Carter. She suffered a recurrence of cancer and died in 1990, at age sixty.

The consensus meeting would not be the last word on screening in the United States. The debate would intensify over the following decades, and the NIH would hold another consensus development conference in 1997. But any hope of resolving differences between those who believed in early detection and those who had doubts would be shattered. Consensus would prove impossible.

Four CONSPIRACY OF HOPE

"Why do you keep putting it off?" a mother asks her daughter in a nagging, exasperated tone, as if they've had the conversation many times before. It's a fleeting moment in a TV ad depicting busy professional women, elegantly dressed and perfectly groomed, rushing through the frame, cancelling appointments, making excuses that they've been meaning to go but just haven't had time. Some of the women look to be in their thirties and some a little older, but the frenetic camera never settles long enough to reveal their ages. After about eight seconds of breathless motion blur, almost devoid of colour, we see that the ad is for GE's breast cancer detection system. What these hectic women keep putting off is a mammogram. An authoritative male voice pronounces in a scolding tone that the GE system can help increase survival of breast cancer to 99 percent. A door in a medical clinic slams ominously, and the final message, in big white letters, flashes onto a dark screen: "A Mammogram. Don't put it off." The ad played on American TV networks in the late 1980s and early 1990s and would have been seen in Canada too. GE Healthcare, a division of General Electric, is one of the world's largest manufacturers of mammography imaging equipment.

In spite of the 1977 consensus development meeting and the recommendation that screening of women under age fifty cease, the American Cancer Society officially recommended, in 1980, that women aged thirty-five to forty should have a "baseline" mammogram. In 1983, it recommended that women between forty and forty-nine have a screening mammogram every one to two years and that women over fifty have a mammogram once every year. The Breast Cancer Detection

Demonstration Project had made mammography a growth industry, and by the time GE's "Don't put it off" campaign rolled out, numerous magazine ads and highway billboard signs were already telling women, "If you don't get a mammogram you need more than your breasts examined" or "Give your mother the gift of life, give her a mammogram for Mother's Day." An American Cancer Society campaign in 1987 told women: "It's essential to have a mammogram" and "A mammogram lets your doctor 'see' breast cancer before there is a lump when the cure rates are near 100%." The American Cancer Society's and GE's claims of such high cure rates were exaggerations, fanciful manipulations of partial data.

Charles Wright wasn't buying any of it. Wright was a young surgeon at the University of Saskatchewan in Saskatoon when the push for mammography screening took hold in the early 1980s. The rhetoric from the American Cancer Society was seeping across the border, Canadian doctors were going to medical conferences where screening was discussed and promoted, and Canadian women were seeing the ads. Wright was a general surgeon with a special interest in breast surgery, and he was noticing "a line" of women appearing for a surgical consultation after a screening mammogram they'd been told would be good for them. "And lo and behold, there was a suspicious lesion on the mammogram," Wright remarks dryly. "What woman is going to be happy to leave it at that and say, oh well, we'll see how it goes?" he asks. So the suspicious lesion would lead to surgery, treatment, and the downstream issues that follow. He began to fear that women might be undergoing unnecessary biopsies and further surgery, while suffering the anxiety all of that entails, for benign disease. He decided to look at the evidence on mammography screening and found it wanting. In 1986, he wrote a paper for the journal *Surgery*, concluding that the harms outweighed the benefits.

That paper made Charles Wright a controversial figure. He didn't mind; he was accustomed to being criticized for unpopular views. Wright immigrated to Saskatoon from Glasgow in 1971 almost by accident. He had done a research fellowship at McGill University in Montreal, where his work led to winning a gold medal from the Royal College of Physicians and Surgeons of Canada. By this time, he was back in Glasgow, but he returned to Canada for the award event, where he happened to meet the head of surgery at the University of Saskatchewan, who promptly offered him a job. He would be an assistant professor and surgeon at University Hospital and would also have his own research facilities. He recalls that the pay was okay too. Wright is wiry and trim with direct blue eyes and a forthright, purposeful demeanour. He still speaks with a no-nonsense Scottish burr that must have been much more pronounced when he moved to Canada, but his accent was not the only reason he stood out in Saskatoon.

In Britain, where Wright trained, breast surgeons had moved away from doing radical mastectomies for cancer. In Saskatoon, he started to think even simple mastectomies were too drastic and began to do lumpectomies, reasoning that minimal surgery would still remove the cancer in the breast, and radiation and chemotherapy would treat the possibility that the cancer had spread. He didn't see how tearing out muscles and lymph nodes could be helpful. Researchers abroad may have been questioning radical mastectomies for many years, but in everyday clinical practice, surgeons in Canada and the United States still preferred them. No one else in Saskatchewan was doing lumpectomies, Wright says. His colleagues did not approve and were so antagonistic that at one point he feared he might even lose his licence because "there was a group that felt this young surgeon from Britain was clearly incompetent, because he wasn't doing the right treatment for breast cancer." He tells this story with some reflective bemusement and suggests that his colleagues ought to have been reading the literature. But at the time, proponents of minimal surgery for breast cancer were lonely pioneers.

It was with the same self-confident questioning of the status quo that Charles Wright tackled the subject of breast screening. In his 1986 *Surgery* paper titled "Breast Cancer Screening: A Different Look at the Evidence," he reviewed the data from the original screening trial, the HIP study in the 1960s, and from the demonstration project a decade later. The demonstration project was not a randomized trial, had no control group, and therefore could offer no information comparing screened women to unscreened women. But it did collect some data on the number of cancers detected and how advanced the cancers were. Wright also looked at a new trial from Sweden published in the *Lancet* in 1985. Mammography screening enthusiasts were touting the Swedish National Board of Health and Welfare Study, also known as the Swedish Two-County trial, as a landmark. It was a large study begun in 1977, with 163,000 women in the counties of Kopparberg and Östergötland enrolled and randomized into two groups, screened and unscreened. The report in the *Lancet* analyzed seven years of data. The results were similar to those from the New York HIP study, indicating a 31 percent reduction in mortality among screened women over age fifty compared to the unscreened control group. But the Swedish study, like the HIP study, also found no reduction in mortality in women aged forty to forty-nine.

When Wright looked at the demonstration project data, he found that 3.58 percent of women screened were referred for surgical consultation and 0.54 percent were found to have cancer, meaning that 3.04 percent had biopsies that turned out to be negative. When he looked at the mortality statistics from the Swedish and HIP studies, he saw that, yes, there did appear to be a 25 to 30 percent reduction in mortality in screened women over fifty. But that's the relative number. To put it in a different context, Wright looked at the absolute number, asking, 25 to 30 percent of what? To figure that out, he looked at the actual number of deaths. Ten-year data from the HIP study found 146 deaths among the 33,000 women in the screened group and 192 deaths in the same number of women in the control group. So there was a difference of forty-six, which is roughly 25 percent of 192. But in absolute numbers, forty-six lives saved out of 33,000 is 0.144 percent of all the women screened. The absolute numbers in the Swedish study revealed an even smaller reduction in mortality, only 0.049 percent in the screened group. Another way to express it, Wright wrote in his paper, was that one in 694 in the HIP study benefited from screening and one in 2,041 benefited in the Swedish study. Calculating that the harm far outweighed the benefits, he wrote that the American Cancer Society's recommendations should be ignored and that only women at high risk for breast cancer should be screened.

Soon after the article's publication, Wright accepted an invitation to a conference on mammography at Johns Hopkins University in Baltimore. He has a vivid memory of what happened. "They had a whole day of people telling this large national audience how wonderful mammography was, then I was there with a contrary opinion, with evidence I thought was fairly strong. I presented this paper which was greeted with a deathly silence, and lots of people were visibly upset." A coffee break followed his talk, and he was standing around, avoided by everyone except the organizer of the conference, "who felt he had to look after me," Wright guesses. Then "a very angry-looking elderly radiologist came up and sort of punched me in the chest with his finger and said 'You don't understand, boy; you've got your hand in our pockets.'" The radiologist needn't have feared for his pockets. Charles Wright continued to speak out about screening, but he was no match for a mammography machine gaining momentum.

In October 1987, an announcement from the White House ensured that the momentum would gather force: Nancy Reagan was about to have surgery for breast cancer. The first lady had had an annual checkup and a screening mammogram. When the nurse who did the mammogram said she needed to do a few x-rays over again, Reagan's stomach knotted. After the additional tests, White House physician John Hutton came into the room with the grim news. "We think we've seen something," he said. "We think it's a tumour of the left breast. We'll need a biopsy." The next day, a cancer specialist told Reagan she had a choice of a lumpectomy to remove the tumour and a little surrounding tissue or a modified radical mastectomy. Even though lumpectomies were becoming popular, she chose the mastectomy, not wanting to interrupt her busy schedule with the weeks of radiation that a lumpectomy would necessitate. Also, she was afraid that she'd never stop fretting about what might have been left behind if they didn't take the entire breast.

Just eleven days after her mammogram, she entered Bethesda Naval Hospital for surgery. The surgeon planned to do a frozen section biopsy first. If the tumour were malignant, he would immediately proceed with a mastectomy. "Please don't wake me to have a conversation about it. Just do it," Reagan commanded.

It turned out that the first lady had a tiny, non-invasive tumour, only seven millimetres in diameter, confined within a milk duct. About the size of a lemon seed, the width of a pencil, it was about the smallest tumour a mammogram could detect. When a White House press briefing released the details, some experts were critical of such an extreme response to so tiny a cancer. Journalist and advocate Rose Kushner, who would have been disappointed that Reagan acquiesced to the one-step mastectomy she'd been fighting so long to stop, accused her of "setting women back ten years." But it was an incredible news story and a triumph for mammography. When asked about the mastectomy, Reagan said the decision felt right for her, but she wasn't trying to influence other women to do the same. She defended it as a feminist choice, hers to make. On the subject of screening, however, she was adamant that every woman should have an annual mammogram beginning at age forty. She became a mammography ambassador, actively participating in an American Cancer Society promotional campaign. Millions of women witnessed a serene Nancy Reagan, perfectly coiffed and wearing a simple grey dress, staring directly at them through their TV screens. She urged them to know one word: mammography. There could not be a more powerful endorsement.

The American Cancer Society was intent on convincing women that with early detection, breast cancer could be almost 100 percent curable, although it had no evidence that was true. Charles Wright took note of its commercials and collected its magazine ads. In an interview for a CBC documentary in 1991, he accused the American Cancer Society of leading a conspiracy of hope. "These are frankly lies which can only be understood, interpreted by the desire to generate this hope and there are certain medical, financial, political implications in all of this too of course." When he gave that interview, Wright had recently moved away from Saskatoon and from surgery to become vice-president of medicine at Vancouver General Hospital. In 1995, he moved into another administrative role as director of the Centre for Clinical Epidemiology and Evaluation at the University of British Columbia. He eventually stopped talking about mammography, frustrated that no one seemed to be listening.

Meanwhile, on the third floor of the McMurrich Building in Toronto, Anthony Miller and Cornelia Baines, along with Teresa To and Claus Wall, the two other scientists leading the Canadian National Breast Screening Study, were approaching the final stages of their massive project. When Charles Wright published his critique of mammography screening in 1986, the Canadian study was already in its sixth year. Recruiting for the study ended in March 1985. Screening would be completed by June 1988, with the majority of the women in the mammography group having five annual screens and a small number having four.

It was right about the time the Canadians finished their recruiting that news came from Sweden's Two-County trial: early detection was apparently reducing breast cancer deaths by 30 percent. The report in the *Lancet* was a scant three-and-a-half pages, but it was the first since the New York HIP study, and it would have a monumental impact. The mammography research community was a small one, so Miller and Baines certainly knew about the Swedish study and were keen to see the results. Miller had met one of its lead investigators, a radiologist named László Tabár. Sometime after his own study got under way, Miller was in Sweden on business for the Union for International Cancer Control. He believed in seeking expert opinion and advice from people who shared his research interests, and Tabár was known for his expertise in doing mammograms and reading them. So Miller took a side trip to Tabár's centre to learn more about the Swedish trial.

When the Swedish results were published, Miller had reservations. He had noted some significant differences between Tabár's study and his. One was the way in which study participants were randomized. In the Canadian study, women were randomized individually in such a way that the researchers could ensure that their screened group and controls were evenly matched in a wide number of specific variable characteristics, such as age, smoking history, weight, level of education, place of birth, occupation, and family history of breast cancer. In the Swedish study, the combined population of the two counties was divided into nineteen blocks. In one county, each block was divided into two units of roughly equal size, with one unit going to the mammography group and the other to the control group. In the other county, blocks were divided into three units, with two units allocated to screening and one to a control group. This method is known as cluster randomization, and the Swedish study accounted for no other variable but age, making it difficult to know whether the groups were well matched. Another difference was that the Canadian study was designed to test the effectiveness of mammography plus physical exam versus physical exam alone in women over fifty. In the Swedish study, mammography was the only form of screening. A third difference was that the Swedish study took only one x-ray view of each breast, whereas the Canadian study took two different views. Finally, in the Swedish study, the screened women were screened once every two to three years. In the Canadian study, screening was done annually.

Miller came away from his visit to Sweden with some concerns about how the Tabár team was analyzing cause of death. It was vital to know whether a woman truly died of breast cancer or whether she had breast cancer but died of something else, such as a heart attack, an infection, or a car accident. Assigning cause of death incorrectly can skew results. Miller had learned from his work with the HIP study that a separate review panel should independently assess deaths. He was, in fact, a death reviewer for that study. The Canadian trial had an independent death review committee. In Sweden, members of local project groups classified the deaths.

When Cornelia Baines saw the Swedish results in the *Lancet*, something jumped out at her. It was the same puzzling thing she had seen in the Canadian data. The younger age group, screened women between forty and forty-nine, experienced slightly more breast cancer deaths than the women who were not screened. As the number of deaths was so few in that age group, it wasn't possible to make firm conclusions, or even inferences, because the difference could be due to nothing more than chance. But that someone else was observing the same odd, inexplicable trend as in the early Canadian results reassured her. More importantly, however, screening was apparently not reducing breast cancer death in women under fifty, at least not in the women who had been followed in the study for seven years. But it was fair and reasonable to suggest, as László Tabár did, that a longer follow-up could yield different data. And although there was no evidence yet that screening benefited women in their forties, he had no doubt that screening older women, aged fifty to seventy-four, was reducing breast cancer death.

Whatever reservations Anthony Miller had about the Swedish study, one thing was clear. Proponents of screening had new ammunition. This was the first major screening trial since the much older HIP study. Now modern mammography, with more precise equipment, was producing the same result. The Swedish Two-County trial told the radiology community, the American Cancer Society, and the imaging industry what they wanted to hear: mammograms save lives. This was the atmosphere in which the Canadian National Breast Screening Study was operating. As they began to sift through their data, Miller and Baines knew if they got different results and found that mammography screening didn't work, no one would listen.

In the 1980s, mammography was a rapidly changing technology. Miller and Baines were epidemiologists, experts in doing clinical trials, but to conduct a trial of mammography, they needed the help of experts in radiology. Miller had been following the Breast Cancer Detection Demonstration Project in the United States and served on a special committee reporting to the 1977 consensus meeting at the NIH. He knew personally many of the radiologists who were considered the best in their field. When the Canadian National Breast Screening Study got under way, its sponsors, the National Cancer Institute of Canada, the Canadian Cancer Society, and Health and Welfare Canada, created a policy advisory group to oversee it. The policy advisory group needed a radiologist, and because Canadian radiology experts would be involved in the study, it was necessary to go to the United States to find independent experts. That, and Miller's own connections, resulted in a succession of highly influential American radiologists, all fervent believers in screening, having privileged access to the Canadian study. Conflict was inevitable.

One of the early advisers was Wende Logan-Young from Rochester, New York, a radiologist who, in 1975, had founded a breast clinic that still exists. It claims to be the first dedicated breast centre in the United States. Logan-Young quit the Canadian study over a dispute about the extent of her role. She complained that she was not allowed to see the mammograms. Baines and Miller say this is not true. She could see the films any time she wished, they explain; they simply didn't want to risk sending boxes of them out of the country. They wanted her to come to Toronto.

Stephen Feig, a professor of radiology at Thomas Jefferson University Hospital in Philadelphia, was the next to come into the advisory group, and he agreed to read films in Toronto, a day ahead of the meetings he would attend every six months. His first concern was the way in which the Canadians were doing the mammograms. When they started in 1980, they did two x-ray views of each breast, in accordance with the standards of the day in North America. One was a view from above the breast, called the craniocaudal view. It is still one of the routine views in screening today. The other was a view taken straight across the side of the breast, the mediolateral view. When Miller set up the protocol for the study, he sought counsel from American radiologist Myron Moskowitz, who led the demonstration project in Cincinnati. According to Miller, Moskowitz advised him to use the mediolateral view because it was the one most widely used in the United States at the time, even though Swedish doctors had developed a modification, the mediolateral oblique view, which allowed radiologists to see more of the upper quadrant of the breast. When Feig became a member of the policy advisory group, he recommended that the Canadian study switch to mediolateral oblique imaging. All the study centres made the change in 1985, except for one in Toronto that had already adopted the mediolateral oblique view some time before.

It was an example of how the Canadian study had to adapt to new technology and new practices as it went along. But even though he'd been on the scene for only a year, Stephen Feig thought the Canadian researchers took too long to heed his advice. Anthony Miller acknowledges that it took a while to persuade every study radiologist to make the change, but he also points out that the mediolateral oblique view was not routinely used in the United States, even by 1983. It marked the beginning of a persistent accusation from American radiologists that the films in the Canadian study were poor. Feig would become one of the study's harshest critics.

It's not that there weren't problems. When the Canadian National Breast Screening Study was set up, Canadian radiologists were accustomed to reading diagnostic mammograms, mammograms performed when a woman or her doctor felt a lump or noticed other symptoms that needed investigation. Screening programs did not yet exist, and radiologists were simply not accustomed to exams of asymptomatic women. They had to learn a new art of assessing women much more quickly than they would in a diagnostic setting. Equipment for modern film-screen mammography, more advanced than the equipment used in the US demonstration project, was the prerequisite for establishing a study screening centre. The study, however, didn't have a budget to buy its own mammography machines. The centres were in provincial cancer hospitals or teaching hospitals across the country, where provincial governments fund the equipment. Most started with new, but one had second-hand equipment. Even new equipment became outdated quickly as technology changed, and several centres needed to upgrade in the later years of the study. The few that didn't were stuck with older machines.

Peter Scholefield, who was the executive director of the National Cancer Institute of Canada at the time and responsible for oversight of the study, remembers a lot of discussion about the quality of the mammograms in the policy advisory group meetings and a continuous effort to improve. But there were growing pains. Two of the three centres that joined the study in 1981 performed poorly at first, either because the films weren't good enough or the radiologist wasn't reading them accurately. One centre made changes quickly; at the other, the original study radiologist had to be replaced before performance improved.

For quality purposes, the study had a built-in protocol for review of the films. At regular intervals, samples were sent to Toronto, to the study's reference radiologist, Douglas McFarlane, to test whether he agreed with the local radiologists' findings. A high level of agreement is an indication of good performance. His job was also to suggest changes if the films weren't good enough. At the same time, the reference physicist, Martin Yaffe, was monitoring the equipment in each centre for technical quality and radiation levels. They could obtain better images with higher radiation exposures, but the goal was to obtain optimal imaging while keeping exposure at an acceptable minimum. Cornelia Baines had the job of communicating the results from the annual reviews to the local centres. Local physicians who had their own ways of doing things didn't always receive the feedback kindly. But in addition to the ongoing review process, the study radiologists and surgeons attended yearly meetings where they looked at films and discussed them in a collegial environment.

For his first assessment as an adviser, Stephen Feig asked for a selection of certain films. He wanted early mammograms from every centre. He wanted mammograms showing severe dysplasia, a term for benign conditions in the breast that include irregular lumps, cysts, and abnormal cells. He wanted films where the centre radiologist had missed the diagnosis. Studying problem mammograms would be instructive, but it also meant that he would see an unrepresentative sample. In an annual meeting, Baines described it as a sample predetermined to be unsatisfactory. Yaffe called it "loaded," although he acknowledged that some of the films could have been better technically.

Feig reviewed sixty mammograms and determined that only half were technically acceptable. Quality depended on the contrast and resolution of images and whether they were too light or too dark. Proper positioning of the breast was also a factor. He made suggestions for ways in which the mammograms could be improved, and Baines passed on his comments to the radiologists in the study centres. In a letter to the chair of the policy advisory group, Feig wrote that he wanted to emphasize the poor quality of the films but thought the problems were easily remedied. He was equally critical in subsequent reviews, and tensions escalated. In January 1986, after assessing three films from each centre, he reported to the policy advisory group that nine out of fifteen centres "had at least one study where the technique was so poor that that there would be a moderate or high chance that a nonpalpable cancer could be missed." He then wrote to Baines to say that the technical quality was not improving and might even be deteriorating. Passing on his review notes to study radiologists, Baines attempted to soften the blow, telling them, "Dr. Feig may be applying standards somewhat unrealistic for the screening context. While this is so, some of his criticisms were very valid." She added that study personnel must be seen to be responding in a reasonable fashion.

The study radiologists became incensed. So did Anthony Miller. He felt that Feig, as an academic working in a specialty environment, had inflated expectations of what was needed in screening and was damaging the goodwill the study had earned from its experienced mammographers. He argued that the cancer detection rate in the study was as good as would be expected in screening, that the standard of mammography in the centres was the best available in Canada, and that great efforts had been made to ensure technical quality. Livid at what he perceived as an accelerating attack, he wrote to Feig, telling him, "You cannot transpose the standards of diagnostic evaluation of abnormalities into the screening situation." Miller emphatically made the point that Feig's insistence on an unreasonable standard would make it impossible to provide screening except in specialized situations. On April 9, 1986, after a year and a half in the job, Feig resigned from the policy advisory group, complaining that he had not received adequate support and cooperation for his efforts.

Miller and Baines feel that the American radiologists misunderstood their role in the policy advisory group. The study's reference radiologist, Doug McFarlane, had the responsibility of ensuring quality control and reviewing films done by radiologists in the centres, and the reference physicist, Martin Yaffe, had the task of monitoring the radiation output of the mammography units and advising on the quality of the images. The radiologists on the advisory group weren't study personnel. "They weren't, in fact, meant to be dealing with us directly," says Baines. "Any concerns they had were to be reported to the advisory group. It was an independent data-monitoring committee. Their role was to interact with other members of the advisory group." Peter Scholefield, to whom Baines and Miller reported, confirms that view. Although the advising radiologists might want to look at some films, their role was not to oversee the work of study radiologists. Their job was to attend meetings of the policy advisory group and make recommendations regarding quality control and technology. "The whole concept of a policy advisory group was to ensure that appropriate established procedures were followed," Scholefield explains. "Full minutes were recorded for every meeting and full verbal and printed background reports were provided. If the investigators had repeatedly failed to follow recommendations from the policy advisory group, the issue would surely have been raised at the next meeting. The minutes of those meetings would have reported such failures, but I have no recollection that such was the case."

Feig's interpretation was that Miller and Baines weren't listening. Yet before he resigned, he was aware that Miller, in his ongoing efforts to ensure quality mammograms, had invited László Tabár to travel from Sweden to attend the annual meeting of study radiologists and surgeons in March of that year. Tabár made a well-received presentation on some of the ways mammography could be improved. When the two days were over, he stayed to review films that Feig had assessed in February, and Cornelia Baines forwarded his comments and suggestions to the centre radiologists. "I'm sure it will be interesting for you to know," she wrote, "that he felt there was a much lower risk of missing an impalpable cancer than has previously been suggested." Miller and Baines both thought Tabár was an excellent teacher.

But Tabár would be no friend of the Canadian study. Only one month after his visit to Toronto, Tabár was back in Canada for a breast cancer symposium in Banff, Alberta, where he told a Canadian Press reporter that he rejected the Canadian trial as a waste of time and money. He questioned the value of comparing the benefits of mammography to physical exams. He said that while Canadian authorities pondered the role that mammograms can play, women were going to die. When Baines quizzed him about the story, he protested that these were the reporter's words, not his, and that his own thoughts were much more complex. "However," he added, "if this is going to help the Canadian radiologists in getting decent technical facilities and creating some balance between the physical examination and mammography arms in the study, the article will have an important function." The idea that the Canadian study expended more effort on well-done physical exams than on upgrading mammography equipment would become a repeated complaint from those who wanted to find fault.

When Stephen Feig departed, the study's sponsors replaced him with another American radiologist. Ed Sickles was a professor of radiology and the chief of breast imaging at the University of California, San Francisco, and a respected authority on mammography. Sickles knew Feig and knew he had resigned. He wasn't keen on stepping in because, he says, he didn't want to be "just another one in a line of people who would suggest things needed to be improved and then nothing would be done." But whoever called him (he doesn't remember who) managed to persuade him that his voice would be heard.

Sickles came to the study with a message. He told the annual meeting of radiologists and surgeons in 1987 that he had done an initial review of their mammograms, and in his opinion, they had improved tremendously compared to the early mammograms. But, he said, criticism from previous reviewers had created a lot of negative comment outside Canada: "You have a very bad press which will have an adverse impact on the National Breast Screening Study results, regardless of outcome." If the results favoured mammograms, he said, people would say they could have been better. If the results indicated that mammography was not great, it would be because the mammograms were bad. Sickles recommended the review of a larger sample of mammograms in order to document the improvements and that such a review be published before the study results were reported. It would be a shame, he said, if American radiologists dismissed the Canadian results. He suspected that the study's mammography was better than what was done in the community and noted that influential radiologists in the United States had an incorrect perception of the mammography standards in the Canadian study.

Anthony Miller was well aware of the American radiologists' prejudgment. So was Cornelia Baines. Miller wanted to deal with the accusations of inferior mammography and agreed with Ed Sickles's recommendation for a review, so he went ahead and designed it. In 1988, Sickles and Miller invited three external reviewers who had not previously been involved in any reviews of the study to take part. They were Daniel Kopans, from the Department of Radiology at Massachusetts General Hospital and Harvard University; Myron Moskowitz, the radiologist from Cincinnati; and Douglas Sanders, a radiologist from Toronto General Hospital. The reviewers would look at a random sample of ten films for each year of the study, from each of the fifteen centres. They would meet in Toronto.

Baines becomes incensed when she recalls what happened. Miller was away, and she was left to deal with the reviewers on her own. They arrived at her home for drinks before going out to dinner and told her, only then, that they would judge all of the films by the standards of 1988 mammography. Stunned, she tried to tell them it didn't seem appropriate to judge mammograms from 1980 by the standards of 1988. There had been big changes in the field. It wasn't what Kopans and Moskowitz had agreed to before coming to Toronto, but they told her that if they couldn't do as they proposed now, they would leave without doing the review. She didn't know what to do. "Now I'd be different," she says. "I would have told them, 'God bless you, go away.' I didn't have the courage to do that. I'd only been on the study for seven years, and these were important people, and they had come from far away, and that was what they were going to do, and I thought, well, we'll have to deal with this later on." The biggest problem with judging the mammograms by 1988 standards was that it predetermined that all of the mammograms done with a mediolateral view instead of the mediolateral oblique view would fare badly.

The review was published in the *American Journal of Roentgenology* in October 1990. Baines and Miller were the lead authors on the paper, and the names of the three reviewers, Kopans, Moskowitz, and Sanders, were also listed, along with Ed Sickles and the two other members of the Canadian study team, Claus Wall and Teresa To. Baines and Miller reported that the films were scored according to four criteria relating to breast positioning, exposure, and image quality. With regard to image quality, only half of the mammograms from the first two years of the study were deemed satisfactory. Image quality improved, however, and by 1985, 68 percent of the mammograms scored satisfactory. By 1986, after the change to the mediolateral oblique view, 85 percent scored satisfactory. When judged by the other criteria, the films scored better. Miller and Baines noted that the review demonstrated the importance of monitoring the quality of mammography in screening programs.

But that was not the end of it. Daniel Kopans, the reviewer from Harvard, did not agree with the paper and in the very same issue published a commentary that essentially dismissed it and the Canadian study. "Because of poor mammography the result of this trial will always be suspect," he wrote. It was odd that a researcher would write such a commentary while leaving his name on the original paper. And odd that the journal would accept it. Kopans admits that it was odd. "How many people write a paper and then say the conclusions are incorrect?" He explains that he left his name on the paper because he did the work, and he wrote the commentary because he disagreed with the interpretation. Miller, having learned about Kopans's commentary in advance, wanted to write a reply in the same issue. Instead, the journal agreed to publish a rebuttal one month later, authored by Miller, Baines, and Sickles. "The discouraging fact that almost 50 percent of the mammograms offered in the first 2 years of screening were judged to be unsatisfactory is perceived in a different light if the reader knows that only 5.1 percent of all the mammograms were produced in the first two years of screening," they wrote. "Only five of the eventual fifteen centres had opened in that period." The review noted that by 1985, only 6 percent of study participants had the complete number of screening mammograms required for the study. Later, Miller regretted that they didn't think to select the films for review differently. Submitting an equal number from each centre meant that the smaller locations had unequal weight in terms of the evaluation, and at least one of those centres was performing poorly. In retrospect, says Miller, the number of films from each centre should have reflected the number of women in the trial.

Today, Ed Sickles is one of the Canadian study's critics and discusses it, and Anthony Miller, in a disdainful, dismissive tone. "It was Dr. Miller's contention throughout that there were no problems with the radiology. He felt he was being unjustly blamed for something he had no control over. It was just the way it was done in Canada and that's the way it should be tested." Sickles also says, "You know, you can't have a lot of respect for a person who is told repeatedly that he's doing something wrong who just doesn't listen, when you're telling him he's doing something wrong in your field, not his field." When reminded that the images improved over the years, Sickles retorts, "That just means he started listening." He also defends Daniel Kopans's unusual commentary. Yet, oddly, Sickles was a signatory, with Miller, to the letter responding to it. He says he doesn't remember that and suggests that his name must have been put there without his knowledge, an allegation that genuinely horrifies Miller. "Oh, come on," he groans. "I would never include somebody on a paper without getting their agreement to what went in." The journal that published the review, the *American Journal of Roentgenology*, says it always contacts co-authors to get agreement for copyright transfer. As for Sickles's contention that Miller just wouldn't listen, Peter Scholefield disputes that. He remembers that Miller did want his study to reflect "the prevailing conditions in the country at the time" and was always ready to make changes to improve the quality of the mammography.

Was the quality of the early mammography in the study a serious problem that would affect the outcome of the study or simply a red herring that radiologists such as Kopans and Moskowitz perpetuated to cast doubt about results they didn't like? By 1990, when the review of the films was published, many in the radiology community already knew the study was not finding benefit from mammography. Radiologists were understandably nervous and skeptical about the Canadian research. They also had confidence in Tabár, one of their own. Cornelia Baines argues that the Canadian study did a better job of identifying tumours. She wonders how, if its mammography was so poor, the Canadian study had higher cancer detection rates than the Swedish study and how the tumours detected in the Canadian study were smaller. The Canadian breast screening trial's openness to scrutiny is unprecedented. No other mammography study had or has invited external review. Baines thinks now they trusted too much. "We were stupid enough to let them do it. We had a very naive conviction that people were scientific and honest and intellectually curious, and we didn't realize that there was going to be only one answer that was acceptable."

Naive? Possibly, but *innocent* is probably a better word. Miller and Baines had every reason to expect a sincere desire to want to know whether screening mammography worked, on the part of everyone involved. That's what the authors of the original New York HIP study wanted, and it's what the consensus development meeting on breast cancer screening wanted too. But by the end of the 1980s, the clamour for screening had become a thunderous roar, driven by the favourable Swedish study, which reported a 30 percent reduction in breast cancer death. The National Health Service in Britain launched a public screening program in 1988. Sweden followed in 1989. In Canada, the Canadian Association of Radiologists was recommending screening programs, and so was the Canadian Task Force on the Periodic Health

Examination. British Columbia established its screening program in 1988; four more provinces launched programs in 1990. The prevailing wisdom was so entirely on the side of breast screening that one study that begged to differ didn't have a chance. Things would change. Eventually, the Swedish study would become the outlier, not the Canadian, but that would take a very long time.

Five   WHEN RADIOLOGISTS ATTACK

Daniel Kopans looks the part of a kindly professor. In a YouTube video from the 2014 annual meeting of the Radiological Society of North America, he is answering questions from the editor-in-chief of AuntMinnie.com, an internet forum for radiologists and related professionals in the imaging industry. *Aunt Minnie* is jargon among radiologists for an x-ray that reveals a perfectly obvious and specific diagnosis. One radiologist might say to another, "Ah, that's an Aunt Minnie!" meaning that the image allows for only one definite conclusion. If it looks like Aunt Minnie, then it's Aunt Minnie. AuntMinnie.com is for insiders, and Kopans's interview is an insider's conversation about breast screening. It's obvious where he stands: the idea that mammography saves lives is an Aunt Minnie.

Kopans is considerably shorter than his questioner, with typical male-pattern baldness, a short grey beard and moustache, and non-descript wire-framed glasses. He's wearing an understated dark suit with a pale blue shirt and red tie, which look to be the same blue shirt and tie he wore for an appearance on a Canadian television program several months earlier. He's slightly rumpled, in a disarming way. He answers the softball questions in a friendly and helpful manner, leaning quietly into the interviewer's hand-held microphone. The controversy over breast screening has been going on too long, he says, longer than the forty years he's been in the field of radiology.

The caption beneath the YouTube video asks, "Is there a conspiracy to stop breast screening?" Kopans believes there is. He tells AuntMinnie.com there is a major effort to try to reduce access to breast cancer screening. "This has involved use of data from trials that were not particularly well done and the analysis of those trials in a non-scientific fashion." He singles out the Canadian National Breast Screening Study as one he argues should not be used in making policy decisions. In the same short conversation, he also denounces a recently published paper in the *New England Journal of Medicine* regarding overdiagnosis of breast cancer. The authors are highly respected epidemiologists, but Kopans dismisses their work, saying the way the paper was done was "faulty," based on "estimates and extrapolations that were incorrect." He alleges that publishing the paper is irresponsible of the *New England Journal of Medicine* and claims that it won't publish anything supportive of screening. He makes the same complaint about the *Annals of Internal Medicine*, the journal published by the American College of Physicians. All of it is signature Kopans: allegations about poorly done trials, faulty analysis, and bias in journals, repeated over and over in his prolific writings, letters to editors, debates, and interviews with journalists. He scatters his accusations liberally, brazenly disregarding scholarly decorum.

Daniel Kopans readily agreed to a request for a telephone interview and sent in advance a long email outlining in detail a timeline, beginning in the 1950s, of what he describes as the issues used to reduce access to screening. He followed up the next morning with a second email adding more to his timeline. He wrote that the "opponents" will "stop at nothing to prove they are correct" and, echoing the AuntMinnie.com conversation, accused those opponents of publishing scientifically unsupportable papers in biased medical journals. Referring specifically to particular health policy academics who have challenged breast screening, he went even further. "There have also been questions raised about who is supporting these groups, and the medical journals," he wrote. "I suspect that the drug companies make money when breast cancers are treated at a later stage."

In the world of breast imaging, Daniel Kopans is an acknowledged leader. He has developed a technique for using x-ray–guided needle biopsies, invented a digital form of 3-D mammography called digital breast tomosynthesis (DBT), published a textbook that is now in its third printing, and authored over 250 journal articles. He holds several patents and served on the medical advisory boards of companies involved in developing imaging equipment. But forty years ago, radiology was not his goal. He describes how he "backed into" the whole field. He grew up in a suburb of Boston, the son of an obstetrician-gynecologist, loving science. He was an anthropology major in college but says he "wasn't smart enough" to be a pure scientist. Wanting to do something socially valuable, he chose medicine. Besides, he hated writing and still does, which, considering the volume of articles he's published in medical journals, not to mention his many letters to editors, is a bit of a joke about himself.

Kopans went to Harvard and thought he might be a surgeon until he realized "that was actually cutting into real people, and that took away the fun." He then thought he could be a pediatrician, but the kids couldn't tell him what was wrong, and the parents couldn't stop talking, so it was frustrating. He fell in love with radiology when he did his residency at Massachusetts General Hospital. "It was fun being able to look inside people and figure out what was going on without actually having to cut them open."

In 1977, his residency completed, he got what he calls a junior staff job in radiology at Massachusetts General. He remembers telling the department's chair he had some interest in laser transillumination of the breast and figures that's what got him the position. Shortly thereafter, the doctor reading mammograms left, and no one else wanted to do them. Kopans describes the chair coming to him in desperation, offering him a position as head of the xeroradiography division if he would agree to take over reading mammograms. So, in 1978, only thirty years old, he became the youngest division head in the history of the hospital. As he became more and more interested in breast imaging and in the possibility of being able to detect small cancers, two mammographers who were leading the field, Ed Sickles and Myron Moskowitz, became his mentors.

Kopans positions himself as someone who almost dropped out of medicine because he didn't feel competent, and as someone who slept through statistics in medical school. Twice when commenting on the work of his "opponents," he said it shouldn't take a "dumb radiologist such as [him]" to point out what's wrong to biostatisticians. Although his speech is sprinkled with "you know" and "I mean," an air of complete confidence in his own rightness contradicts the conceit of humility. He isn't shy about saying he is one of the world's experts in breast cancer screening. He represents himself as someone who above all wants to tell the truth. "It may sound stupid, but I'm an honest person. I know what's gone on over the years, and I don't think we should be lying to women and their physicians. I don't want to use the word *lying*, but it's become lying."

Kopans declares that those opposed to screening are people who play with the data and write papers in the *New England Journal of Medicine* "that are just scientific hoaxes." In the scientific world, the usual approach to disagreement is to say, "I don't agree with your conclusions, and here is some data that you might also consider." That's not Kopans's style and never has been. He is famously combative. A 1997 article in *Science* by Gary Taubes anonymously quoted scientists who described Kopans's tactics as "intellectual terrorism" or "scientific McCarthyism." A director of the NCI told *Science* Kopans employs "a pattern of inflammatory, accusatory approaches that are antithetical to the requirements of scientific discourse." Anthony Miller's and Cornelia Baines's experiences are testimony to that assessment. Since the day that Kopans was invited to review the films in the Canadian National Breast Screening Study, he has not missed a chance to criticize their work. Less than a year after publishing his critique of the quality of the films in their study, Kopans found another opportunity to denounce them.

The front-page headline was stunning: "Women Who Have Breast Scanning Are More Likely to Die of Cancer." It was June 2, 1991. One of the world's biggest newspapers, London's *Sunday Times*, had somehow acquired preliminary results from the Canadian breast screening trial. Its story broke the news that, among the women aged forty to forty-nine in the study, a greater number in the screened group died than in the unscreened control group. Miller never learned who leaked the information, but he had discussed some preliminary results at the International Cambridge Conference on Breast Cancer Screening two months earlier. This was not unusual; scientists routinely present preliminary results at conferences.

The *Sunday Times* did not have any statistics, and neither Miller nor Baines would give any when asked. But they confirmed in interviews that they had seen more deaths in the screened women. They had been observing the trend for a while, and it was an open secret among the many people associated with the study. But although the finding was inexplicable and troubling, it was far from conclusive. A headline suggesting that screening was a direct and definite cause of death was entirely misleading and, in Baines's view, sensationalistic. Unavoidably, however, the story spread, as did condemnation of the study. "Doctors Say Breast Scan Study Flawed," read a *Sunday Telegraph* headline on June 9, 1991. That story quoted from Daniel Kopans's earlier dissident commentary in the *American Journal of Roentgenology*: "Unfortunately enormous amounts of time, effort and expense have gone into the Canadian trial. The fact is that because of the poor mammography the results of this trial will always be suspect."

Cornelia Baines told the *Sunday Times* reporter, "Our results are going to be, without question, extremely unwelcome. There is going to be a major outcry." She understood how much was at stake for those who wanted mammography to work. And she was right: there would be an outcry. It would be eighteen months before the Canadian study was finally published, but the anticipated results had already created an international furor. The national breast screening program in Britain was still new, and if women didn't participate, it would fail. The program leaders swiftly latched on to Kopans's view. In a letter to the editor of the *Sunday Times*, the national coordinator of the British screening program wrote: "The Canadian study is significantly flawed on quality grounds" and "much of the research appears to be highly questionable." According to the *Sunday Telegraph*, British doctors reacted with horror, worried that the news was going to scare women off from screening even if they were over fifty, the age at which screening was offered in the United Kingdom.

That reaction magnified when, on June 29, 1991, the *Lancet*, in direct response to the *Sunday Times*, hastened to publish an unsigned editorial. It took an even-handed approach to the Canadian study, but only after first outlining some of the controversy over the quality of the films and the state of the equipment in Canada, referencing Daniel Kopans. The editorial pointed out that the study protocol and the reliability of the data had already been fiercely criticized and added that in the first two years of study, over 50 percent of the mammograms were inadequate. "Only in the last two years of the trial was image quality technically acceptable in more than 70% of screenings." The editorial went on to say that modern equipment was not routinely available at the study centres, and there was no coordinated training program for either radiologists or radiographers.

More positively, the editorial noted that "poor quality mammography may lead to a poor quality screening program but this should not in itself lead to increases in the mortality in the study [screened] group." Other published studies had shown trends in the same direction, it acknowledged, and the death rates in the Canadian study might fall with time. "A longer period of follow-up seems to diminish the adverse effect of mammography in this age group [forty to forty-nine]." No evidence existed, the editorial concluded, to support the introduction of screening mammography for women under fifty.

Anthony Miller promptly responded to the *Lancet* with a reminder that the data were preliminary and said he did not know where the *Sunday Times* got its information. In response to comments about poor-quality mammograms, Miller emphasized that in the first two years, only 5 percent of all the mammograms had been done. A month later, the *Lancet* published a rebuttal from Kopans. He insisted that the mammography was poor, with 15 percent judged unsatisfactory even by the fourth year of screening. But Kopans was counting only the mammograms reviewed. Miller was counting the total number of films in the study.

In that same letter, Kopans introduced a whole other issue that would eventually become the source of even more argument. He said it was his "understanding" that the women who died of breast cancer in the screened group had advanced disease at the time they were diagnosed. He hinted that if there were more advanced cancers in the screened group, perhaps there were problems with the way the women were randomized. Kopans was either speculating about data that he did not have or was inappropriately referencing and abusing inside information. Either way, he fomented rumours. The study was not yet published, yet he raised a series of questions that, just in the asking, cast a shadow on the Canadian trial. Maybe, he speculated, women had a false sense of security after their mammograms didn't show anything and ignored symptoms, thus delaying their treatment. He reasoned that perhaps the false sense of security was the most likely reason for the study's findings, made all the worse by poor-quality films. Ironically, after expressing his own theoretical suppositions, Kopans asserted that the "investigators should avoid incomplete presentation of their data that does not permit objective review. Speculation about the reasons for their findings is dangerous and may result in women avoiding a test that may be life-saving."

The bombshell in the *Sunday Times* was still reverberating in America a year later. In June 1992, the *Journal of the National Cancer Institute* published a story headlined "Author of Canadian Breast Study Retracts Warnings," suggesting that Miller was now retracting the data. The press had already reported that by now, after twelve months of additional follow-up, the excess deaths in women aged forty to forty-nine who'd had mammography had become fewer in number. The number of deaths in the control group was catching up. Still, the fear of mammography the *Sunday Times* generated resulted in "a flood of inquiries" to the NCI, the American Cancer Society, and other medical organizations. Those organizations, "powerless to discuss unpublished data," according to the *Journal of the National Cancer Institute*, "can do little but reaffirm the widely supported recommendation for women in this age group; an annual clinical breast exam and a mammogram every one to two years." It would have been more accurate to call that recommendation widely debated rather than widely supported, but the subtlety was overlooked.

The radiologists quoted in the article didn't seem to get the nuance either. They believed the Canadian study was going to scare women off mammograms, and they wanted to be out in front of the controversy. "Every time there is a headline in the newspaper saying 'Canadian study shows mammography danger to women under fifty' we have to recoup our support," protested Linda Warren, one of the founders of the breast screening program in British Columbia. The article named Warren as one of a "chorus" of radiologists complaining about the quality of the mammograms but did not mention that her program started out in the very clinic at the BC Cancer Agency that had been the Vancouver centre for the breast-screening study, using equipment purchased, new, toward the end of the screening period. Myron Moskowitz, the radiologist who advised Anthony Miller at the beginning of the study, was quoted as saying, "We're left with a study that can be applicable only to a certain situation — the evaluation of poor quality mammography."

Miller fired off a letter in response. He started with the headline. Characterizing his reassessment as a "retraction" certainly was odd. It was as if he had changed his mind, not that the outcome had changed over time. "It is not clear how I can retract a warning I never issued," he wrote. He added that, unfortunately, neither the *Sunday Times* nor the *Lancet* chose to publish the caveats he had "carefully stated when [he] discussed, at what [he] had believed to be a private meeting, some of the preliminary data." Then, in a convincing chronology of the events up to that point, he took direct aim at Myron Moskowitz. Miller was an epidemiologist, not a radiologist, and when he set up the study, he relied on Moskowitz's expertise for advice on protocol. Now Moskowitz, and others, were using this advice against him. "It is clear that screening for women aged forty to forty-nine years will remain controversial," Miller concluded, "while those in authority deny the science."

Daniel Kopans, with his prolific pen, jumped in to counter Miller. "It is indeed unusual to have so much discussion concerning material that has not yet been published," he acknowledged before riffing on an earlier theme. "Irresponsibly suggesting that mammography was detrimental, they ignored the fact that their poor-quality mammography could exacerbate delays in diagnosis" in women who had a false sense of security after a negative screen. Miller had written that he had respect for Kopans as a radiologist but not for his failure to understand statistics. Kopans fired back that Miller's lack of understanding of radiography was at the heart of his study's problems. The rancour ran deep. But Kopans's real concern was how US policy-makers would view the Canadian research.

Screening was the subject of fierce debate in America at precisely this time. In the midst of the controversy over the Breast Cancer Detection Demonstration Project, the NCI issued guidelines meant to put a stop to screening women under fifty. The 1977 consensus meeting reinforced that position with its conclusion that there was no evidence to support screening women in their forties. The American Cancer Society, however, had never really accepted that outcome. In 1983, the society distanced itself completely from the NCI and issued a recommendation that women aged forty to forty-nine undergo screening every one to two years. The American College of Radiology had been making a similar recommendation since 1977 and re-emphasized it in 1982. In an effort to resolve the inconsistencies in screening guidelines, the college, in 1988, initiated a roundtable of interested medical organizations, including the NCI. A year later, in 1989, the roundtable published guidelines recommending mammograms every one to two years for women under fifty and every year for women over fifty. NCI officials, persuaded to change their minds, joined in with ten other organizations that included the American Cancer Society, the American Medical Association, the American Society of Internal Medicine, and four different radiology groups as signatories. Still, in spite of this alliance, there was no nationwide consensus. The American College of Physicians did not join in, maintaining, as it had since 1985, that screening women under age fifty was not advisable. The influential US Preventive Services Task Force, a body set up by the federal Public Health Service five years before the roundtable to scientifically review medical evidence, recommended against screening women under fifty. The efforts to achieve consistency failed. Screening guidelines were all over the place. It was a mess.

The women affected by all of this were not reading the academic journals, the endless arguments, and the nuanced detail. Nor would they have any idea of the personalities driving those arguments. They would have formed opinions based on what they heard in the media or from their doctor. Or they would have thrown up their hands in despair, not knowing what to do. The debate raged in the *Journal of the National Cancer Institute* and in the daily press.

"Doubts Increase on Need for Early Mammogram," headlined a March 1988 *New York Times* story by Gina Kolata, reporting on a review in the *Journal of the American Medical Association*. "New Study Expands Evidence on Benefits of Mammograms," suggested the *Washington Post* in September of that same year, when a new analysis of the old HIP study appeared in the *Journal of the National Cancer Institute*. On July 4, 1989, the headline for another *Washington Post* story on the round-table agreement read: "Mammogram Recommendation Draws Fire." In September 1989, First Lady Barbara Bush made news when she let it be known at the Women's Leadership Summit on Mammography that she had annual mammograms and urged all other women to do the same.

Understandably, a proponent such as Daniel Kopans would find the Canadian study threatening in such an uncertain and volatile environment. Besides, surveys indicated that fewer than half of women over fifty were getting mammograms. In his letter to the *Journal of the National Cancer Institute*, Kopans challenged health policy-makers around the world to consider not the size of the Canadian study but the expertise of breast imagers. "The flaws in the National Breast Screening Study must be taken into account before its results are used to withdraw potentially life-saving access to women at these ages," he wrote. Twenty-two years later, his message in the AuntMinnie.com interview is almost exactly the same.

The politics of breast screening created headlines in Canada too. "Screening of Breasts Called Futile," trumpeted the *Vancouver Sun* a few weeks after the controversial front-page *Sunday Times* story. "Debate Rages Over Study on Breast Cancer," headlined an article in the *Toronto Star* in August 1991. And the following month in the *Montreal Gazette*: "Unpublished Breast-Cancer Study Sparks Furor."

The *Toronto Star*'s article hinted at a rift in the Canadian cancer establishment. The paper reported that "preliminary results of a massive multi-million dollar Canadian study have reportedly shown that for women aged forty to forty-nine, mammograms have no benefit, and may do harm." Interviewed for the story, Miller explained that he'd come up with an answer that people were not prepared to accept, "so they'll attack the study, the technology. It is unacceptable to radiologists; they don't want to see the results. People say if you publish what you know people won't come and be screened. Well, maybe some should not come and be screened." The *Star* reporter also interviewed Peter Scholefield, who had just stepped down as director of the National Cancer Institute of Canada. Scholefield said Miller's discussion of the results before they were published was unethical. "This country is about to embark on an 80 million dollars a year screening program," Scholefield told the reporter. "There are tremendous stakes involved here."

The stakes were high indeed. Organized breast screening had become part of public health policy in Canada. Every year, about five thousand Canadian women were dying of breast cancer. Breast cancer experts and advocates had faith in early detection, just as Miller had before he embarked on his study. In March 1988, twenty-eight representatives from government, professional, and voluntary groups participated in the National Workshop on the Early Detection of Breast Cancer. The Canadian Cancer Society, the Department of National Health and Welfare, and the National Cancer Institute of Canada sponsored the workshop on behalf of the provinces. The workshop met for two days to review the evidence. Its task was to develop a Canadian position on screening. Anthony Miller was among the twenty-eight in the group. So was Cornelia Baines. Peter Scholefield was also at the table, along with prominent radiologists and oncologists. They recommended that women aged fifty to sixty-nine should be offered, and encouraged to participate in, an early detection program that included mammography, a physical breast exam, and the teaching and monitoring of breast self-examination every two years, at dedicated screening centres. The group decided that the evidence to justify screening women in their forties was insufficient.

Contrary to the workshop's recommendations, British Columbia's screening program offered mammograms to women beginning at age forty. Alberta, Saskatchewan, Ontario, and Yukon established screening programs in 1990, and Nova Scotia followed in 1991, offering screening to women aged fifty to sixty-nine every two years. In 1991, ninety thousand Canadian women took advantage of the breast clinics. The new screening programs had a lot invested in making that number grow. The 1991 *Sunday Times* report stating that women who have breast screening were more likely to die of breast cancer was certainly not going to help the cause of the breast screening programs. Rumours about what the Canadian National Breast Screening Study was finding were a threat, and it didn't matter that most of the controversy revolved around mammography for women in their forties. Despite the nationally recommended policy to screen women aged fifty to sixty-nine, many in Canada believed screening should begin earlier. The Alberta, Yukon, and Nova Scotia screening programs, for instance, accepted women in their forties though they did not actively recruit them. The American Cancer Society had long been advocating a "baseline" mammogram at age thirty-nine or forty, and that message reached Canadian doctors, who felt it was a sensible practice.

This, then, was the highly charged atmosphere in which Miller and Baines prepared to publish their long-awaited first results. The mammography industry was poised to denounce the study and the Canadian researchers. Daniel Kopans had already succeeding in casting doubt about the study's validity, and Miller and Baines would soon find they had harsh critics at home. One of them was Martin Yaffe.

Six   A DISSENTER WITHIN

The four pictures hanging side by side, each about a metre by two-thirds of a metre, appear to be sketches, with random scatterings of pinks, greens, purples, and blues thrown onto the canvas among black lines and white streaks. But these are not works of abstract art. Martin Yaffe is giving a tour of the lab where he does his breast imaging research, at Sunnybrook Health Sciences Centre in Toronto. The striking images decorating the lab's entrance are pathology slides, blown up and printed, all pictures of the same breast tumour. The colours are stains injected into the cells to highlight different receptors — the estrogen receptor, for instance — that give clues to the best treatment options. It's astonishing how something so ugly to think about can be so beautiful to look at. For Yaffe, the beauty that he beholds is in the possibility of getting better control of breast cancer. It has occupied most of his life's work.

Yaffe is a senior scientist at the Sunnybrook Research Institute and one of the project leaders in its Breast Cancer Research Centre. It's late on a Thursday afternoon, at the end of summer, just before Labour Day weekend. The labs are quiet. The scientists and technicians are either still on vacation or have gone for the day. Just returned from two weeks at a cottage, Yaffe is relaxed and casual. He is dressed for the record-high temperatures in a short-sleeved blue shirt, beige chinos, and running shoes. His office is a comforting clutter of scientific papers and journals piled high everywhere you look. Four half-empty water bottles peek out from the stacks on his desk. Yaffe has greying hair — a lot of it. His frame is a little soft around the edges; his smile is friendly. He is welcoming and happy to talk.

Casualness is not what you expect from a scientist of his stature. Martin Yaffe is one of the world's leading experts in breast imaging. He is one of the inventors of digital mammography, and in 2015, he was awarded the Order of Canada for his work on developing the technology. He has also done research with 3-D imaging, known as tomosynthesis, the advanced form of mammography that Daniel Kopans developed. Yaffe is currently collaborating with oncologists and cell biologists to see if imaging and pathology can join forces to gain a deeper understanding of cancer tumour biology. He has published hundreds of papers and travelled the world as a speaker and consultant.

In 1978, when Anthony Miller was planning the Canadian National Breast Screening Study and seeking funds for it, Yaffe was completing his PhD in medical biophysics at the University of Toronto. He had come to Toronto from Winnipeg to study and work with his mentor, Harold Johns, a Canadian physicist who had developed cobalt-60 radiation therapy at the University of Saskatchewan in the 1950s, before becoming head of the physics division at the Ontario Cancer Institute and Princess Margaret Hospital in Toronto. Yaffe became a researcher at the hospital and grew interested in mammography when a radiologist colleague asked the physics team to measure the amount of radiation involved. "When I saw how high the doses were and how poor the pictures were," he recalls, "it motivated me to direct my interests into trying to improve the quality of mammography and to do it with less radiation."

Miller, also concerned about radiation in mammography and having to fend off critics who said mammography would cause cancer, approached Johns to help him quantify the radiation. Johns handed the task over to his young protege, and Yaffe became the reference physicist for Miller's study. His job was to monitor the mammography equipment and radiation at each of the study centres. He also saw it as an opportunity to work on improving the quality of the x-ray images, to give the radiologists better tools to work with. He developed a set of physics tests using artificial objects that simulated the breast to measure the sharpness of the image, contrast, and brightness levels, as well as radiation. Part of his role, he says, was to develop some standard of quality across the fifteen sites in the study. He travelled to each centre but did most of his work at Princess Margaret Hospital, analyzing films mailed to him. He worked closely with the study's reference radiologist, Douglas McFarlane, and got to know all of the radiologists brought in as advisers. Although the study required him only part time, Yaffe was an important member of the team. Meanwhile, he was gaining expertise and beginning to experiment with a digital alternative to film mammography. He published his first paper on digital mammography in 1985.

Yaffe's contribution to the study was technical. It wasn't his job to look at the mammograms from a clinical point of view, to decide whether or not something looked like cancer. He's not a medical doctor. The radiologists interpreted the films. But Yaffe had opportunities to observe and learn from them. He sat in the back of the room when Cornelia Baines presented a stack of films to one of the external radiology consultants. Yaffe grew to understand what the radiologists were looking for and how better imaging could help them. Each year, he presented a report to the annual meeting of study radiologists and surgeons.

Once the screening phase of the study ended in 1988, Yaffe's role as the technical expert ended. But by this time, he says, he already wanted to distance himself from the study. He had concerns about the quality of the mammograms. In 1990, when the formal review of the films was published in the *American Journal of Roentgenology*, Daniel Kopans's dissenting commentary reinforced Yaffe's concerns. And by the time Miller and Baines published their first results, Yaffe had aligned himself with the American radiologists who were denouncing them. Even so, academic propriety should have applied and what Yaffe did was unorthodox. The *Canadian Medical Association Journal* was to publish two papers by Miller and Baines on November 15, 1992. Two days in advance, the National Cancer Institute of Canada, the study's sponsor, held a press conference. There had been much rumour and speculation, and there were now huge investments in screening. This would be a big story.

The first of the two papers reported the findings for women aged forty to forty-nine, where half of the fifty thousand women received annual mammograms and physical breast exams and half were controls, assigned to usual care. After seven years of follow-up, the researchers found no difference in mortality between the two groups. This result, already leaked months earlier and much discussed, was as expected. The second paper reported the seven-year findings in women aged fifty to fifty-nine, where half of the forty thousand women in the group were given annual mammograms plus physical breast exams and half received annual physical exams only. The conclusion here was more surprising. In the older age group, the addition of mammography did not have any impact on mortality. The much-wanted proof that screening worked was simply not evident in the data. The results indicated the exact opposite. Screening was not saving lives.

Martin Yaffe was at the press conference. He wasn't listed as an author on either of the two papers, but the director of the National Cancer Institute of Canada, the study's main sponsor, invited him to take a place at the head table. Yaffe wasn't sure he wanted to take part since he didn't agree with the study results, but after some persuading, he acquiesced. "At one point," he recalls, "there was an opportunity for me to say something, and I just basically made the point that I was concerned that there were some major problems with image quality that certainly cast doubts, in my view, as to whether the results of the study were credible."

His comment apparently escaped the media's notice. Yaffe thought it was odd that the press would ignore a comment so divergent from the message of the press conference, odd that the media didn't pick up on the lack of harmony within the team. And then a month later, the *Journal of the National Cancer Institute* published a piece that made him look like a supporter of the study. Yaffe's picture appeared along with Miller's, and Yaffe was reported to have said, "While 1992 mammography equipment was vastly superior to some of the equipment used in the study, the results remain valid." It wasn't at all what he thought, and on top of that, the journal spelled his surname incorrectly, with a double *e*.

Yaffe asked for a retraction. In January 1993, the journal published a correction, quoting him. "The conclusion regarding validity was made not by me, but by Dr. Miller," he said. "In fact I do not share this belief with him, and in my work as reference physicist to the NBSS [National Breast Screening Study], [I] identified many concerns regarding the quality of mammography carried out in some of the screening centres." He listed problems with both equipment and technique and suggested that the only responsible conclusion was that "there is not yet sufficient power to test whether the mortality reduction for which the study was designed actually exists." Daniel Kopans remembers being "aghast" when he saw the comments originally attributed to Yaffe, whom he considered a good friend. With the retraction, Yaffe made sure that everyone knew where he stood. He secured his place in a clique of critics that, along with Kopans, included Stephen Feig, Myron Moskowitz, and Ed Sickles, all American radiologists who had played a role in the Canadian study.

But if publicly disavowing the study at the press conference was a provocative faux pas, so, too, was Miller's failure to name Yaffe as a co-author of the two papers. In addition to the four named authors listed beneath the titles of the papers were, in small print on the front page, the names of over one hundred surgeons, radiologists, and pathologists who were study investigators. Yaffe's name wasn't on that list either. He received a mention only in the final paragraphs, where consultants and advisers were acknowledged and where Miller also acknowledged the reference radiologist, Douglas McFarlane. Miller regrets the slight. He feels it was a mistake not to invite Yaffe to be a co-author of the papers, one he's had to live with since. They have never spoken about it.

Miller doesn't remember exactly what Yaffe said at the press conference. Cornelia Baines doesn't either, recalling vaguely that "he was a fly in the ointment." But she agrees it was wrong to leave Yaffe off the authors list. She reflects ruefully that they may have thought at the time that a technical role in a study didn't merit authorship, and she feels that Yaffe had a justifiable grievance. "It was unfortunate," she says, "because we made an enemy." And Yaffe? If he ever felt aggrieved, he's not admitting it. Today, he says he's glad he wasn't an author on the study. Considering his declared disapproval, it's not surprising; it's consistent with his desire to disassociate. And he certainly did become an enemy. His criticisms became even more severe in later years.

Yaffe says his concerns about the mammograms deepened as the study progressed. Baines doesn't remember having any sense of that. Yaffe's annual reports didn't reveal any particular unease about the quality of the films. As the person responsible for their technical quality, he commented on what needed improvement and how that could be achieved, as required. His tone was professional and encouraging. For instance, in his 1985 report, he wrote that he was generally "quite pleased with both radiation doses and image quality throughout the study." Today, Yaffe describes feeling inhibited about speaking out: "I was very young, I was basically a fresh PhD at the time, I didn't have much clout." Miller, in contrast, was a senior scientist, internationally known. Yaffe knew physics but not cancer, and it took a while, he says, to have enough confidence in his observations to voice his concerns.

If Yaffe's press conference comment went unnoticed at the time, it might have been because it was a mere sidebar to the main event. In 1992, the mantra of early detection was entrenched. Doctors had drilled "early detection is your best protection" into women's brains, and now Canada's National Breast Screening Study was saying, no, it's not. This was an affront to decades of belief and millions of faithful followers. Breast screening doesn't save lives? How could that possibly be true?

Even Miller wasn't entirely convinced. In spite of the results he published, he wasn't ready to give up on screening women in their fifties. Not yet. The Canadian study was consistent with others that had reported no reduction in mortality among women in their forties, but it was alone in its finding that for women in their fifties, mammography was not making a difference when compared to physical breast exams. Miller thought that could change with longer follow-up. Still, the study rankled those radiologists in Canada who insisted on a policy of screening women in their forties and unnerved the new provincial breast screening programs, which feared that women in their fifties would abandon them. Miller and Baines's findings set off an avalanche of controversy.

Danielle Perrault, head of Ontario's breast screening program, and Richard Schabas, the province's chief medical officer of health, rushed to get out a message that would reassure women. It's generally accepted that for population screening to work, the uptake must be at least 70 percent. Possibly fewer than half of Ontario women in their fifties were taking advantage of the program, and they were worried. Perrault and Schabas wrote a widely circulated commentary, "Breast Cancer Screening — Making Sense Out of Confusion." The benefit for women aged forty to forty-nine is unclear, they acknowledged, but promised that "early detection is effective in women 50 years and over." They said the Canadian study was at odds with other studies: six studies involving more than six hundred thousand women had shown that breast cancer deaths could be reduced "up to" 40 percent. But this statistic was a generalization that didn't tell women what 40 percent meant because it didn't tell them the number of actual deaths. It was a use of numbers designed to exaggerate. Was that 40 percent reflected in all studies or just one? Which one? As for women over fifty, comparison to other studies was not entirely fair. The Canadian study was the only one that compared mammography plus physical exams to physical exams alone. The other studies compared screening to no screening. It's not a subtle point.

A debate in the *Canadian Medical Association Journal* ensued. Toronto epidemiologist Antoni Basinski fully endorsed the study. "The initial results of the NBSS do not support regular screening for breast cancer with mammography at any age, but they do provide the opportunity for a rethinking of screening for breast cancer," he wrote in an editorial. He addressed the image quality issue, citing research that had found that the centres' radiologists were skilled at detecting cancer and that their mammography found more cancers than did physical exams. He observed: "Suboptimal quality may be expected to diminish the size of the potential effect, but not abolish it." In an article headlined "When considering attacks against the National Breast Screening Study, consider the sources," physician and journalist Brian Goldman wrote: "The first sounds heard following the study's release was [*sic*] the rush of vested-interest groups anxious to attack it." Goldman found the vehemence of the critics troubling.

On the other side of the debate, Linda Warren, executive director of the screening program in British Columbia, wrote a letter to the editor listing reasons why she thought the study offered no evidence that women shouldn't be screened starting at age forty. Another BC radiologist, H.J. Burhenne, wrote: "Nothing new has been shown at this time, particularly given the poor mammographic technique. Our data in British Columbia show we should continue screening women under the age of fifty." A third letter from Quebec trotted out the poor-quality argument, claiming, "The NBSS is incapable of detecting any reduction in death rates as a result of screening."

The release of the study generated a flurry of media activity. Quebec's association of radiologists called a press conference to condemn the study as "seriously flawed." The Ontario Medical Association declared in the *Toronto Star* that women aged fifty to sixty should not be deterred from screening. "The study could be dangerously misleading," BC surgeon and screening advocate Patricia Rebbeck told the *Province*. Howard Seiden, a Toronto physician and medical columnist, analyzed the study in detail in the *Toronto Star* and *Hamilton Spectator*. He bawled out the study's critics. "A lot of what is going on has nothing to do with science," he argued. "It's simply dirty politics." In Ottawa, the federal government announced the formation of an expert panel to review breast screening policy in light of the study's results.

The ripples of censure spread throughout the United States, where screening was even more controversial than in Canada. Some samples from the headlines illustrate the impact. *Los Angeles Times*: "Mammogram Benefits Questioned in Study." *Chicago Sun-Times*:

"Mammography No Lifesaver, Study Reports." The *Oregonian*: "Canadian Study Raises Doubts About Value of Mammograms." *Chicago Tribune*: "Value of Mammograms Questioned." *Newsday*: "Controversy on Mammography, Canadian Study Questions Benefit." The *Salt Lake Tribune*: "Controversial Canadian Research Questions Mammography's Value." *Los Angeles Daily News*: "A New Canadian Study Has Cast a Shadow Over US Recommendations That Women Ages 40-49 Get Regular Mammograms." The *Washington Post*: "Doubts About Mammograms." All of these articles in the US media got the attention of radiologists, and in the intense days following the publication of the study, Anthony Miller and Cornelia Baines had to bear their wrath. Baines would pick up her phone to hear an anonymous voice, bristling with contempt, call her a murderer.

Behind the scenes, Daniel Kopans and Stephen Feig fomented the ire of their colleagues. They had prepared a briefing memorandum for the American College of Radiology to give doctors tips on how to respond to questions from the media. The memo listed all of their criticisms, but really it was about a fight against any influence the Canadian research might have on US public policy decisions.

The arguments played out in the scientific journals too. But in those, Miller and Baines had allies in like-minded epidemiologists who shared their perspective. Among them were Suzanne Fletcher and her husband Robert Fletcher, the editors of the influential *Annals of Internal Medicine*. They had Canadian connections, having been on the faculty at McGill University's medical school earlier in their careers, and she was also a member of the Canadian Task Force on the Periodic Health Examination. That organization, since renamed as the Canadian Task Force on Preventive Health Care, was created to develop national guidelines for doctors. Two weeks after the breast-screening study was published, the Fletchers plunged into the debate with an editorial titled "The Breast Is Close to the Heart."

The point that emerges most strongly in the Fletchers' editorial is that the Canadian trial wasn't saying anything much different from any other trial, especially regarding women under fifty. The Canadian results were based on seven years of follow-up. The Swedish Two-County trial led by László Tabár had recently reported the same results after eleven years of follow-up. Another smaller study in Sweden and one in the United Kingdom also had failed to show any benefit to screening women under fifty. "Regardless of the reasons for the findings in all these studies, the simple fact is that a universal hope has not stood up to scientific scrutiny," the Fletchers wrote. Even if the critics were right about poor-quality mammograms in the Canadian trial, they argued, that "would be unlikely to nullify completely, any mortality benefit." Regarding women over fifty, the results in the Canadian study were surprising, they noted, and were likely to be just as controversial. This was the first time a randomized trial had compared two different screening modalities — mammography plus physical exam and physical exam alone — and the Fletchers asked, "Can fingers be taught to be as good as mammography?" They suggested that instead of blaming the result on poor-quality mammograms, critics should consider that the results might be due to high-quality physical examinations.

The ruthless politics knew no borders. The fight in the United States continued to make life difficult for Miller and Baines. And then, just when it didn't seem that further bad publicity could be possible, Martin Yaffe broadsided them with another unprecedented attack. Harvard's Daniel Kopans had hinted at issues with randomization, even before the Canadian results were published. When the data became available, Yaffe picked apart the tables and came up with what he thought was evidence that Kopans was right. To this day, he says that what he considers a randomization problem bothers him more than any image quality issues. In a paper he and his colleagues authored in December 1993, in the journal *Radiology*, Yaffe zeroed in on the numbers in the results for women aged forty to forty-nine.

Here's how the randomization worked. When a woman came in to one of the study centres, she signed a consent form, and a nurse performed a clinical exam of her breasts. The nurse then handed the woman over to the centre's coordinator, who assigned her to either the mammography group or the unscreened, usual care group. The coordinator entered the names on one of two allocation lists, on the next available slot on each list in turn, according to five-year age blocks. The women were slotted without regard to the outcome of the clinical exam, and the nurse examiners did not see the lists. If the nurse found a lump in the physical exam, the woman would see the study surgeon for further review.

Among the women under fifty, twenty-five thousand were in the mammography group and twenty-five thousand were in the control group. The study characterized invasive cancers detected in either group by the number of lymph nodes involved: none, between one and three, and four or more. The initial screen, by either mammography or the clinical exam given to all of the women, resulted in an uneven distribution of the women who had four or more lymph nodes involved. Nineteen such women were in the mammography group, and five were in the control group. Yaffe asked how that could be. The number should be equal in both groups. Even more puzzling: among the nineteen women in the mammography group with extensive nodal involvement, only two had cancers detected by mammography alone. Seventeen had cancers palpable in a physical exam. Yaffe argues that, in theory, a nurse or coordinator who felt sorry for a woman with a lump could make sure she was assigned to the mammography group. He can't say anyone actually did that, only that "the data are very much consistent with that happening." And even if the number of women with advanced cancers is small, he says the imbalance would bias the study.

Miller and Baines think this is absurd. There could be no motivation for subverting the randomization. Any woman in the study who was found to have a lump in her breast would have received proper care: a referral to the centre's review clinic, where a study surgeon would determine the necessary diagnostic procedures, including biopsy, fluid aspiration, or diagnostic mammography. The woman's family physician would also have been notified. No coordinator would have any reason to deliberately place a study volunteer into the mammography group.

But things escalated in 1995. A biostatistician at the NCI published a review that reinforced Yaffe's theory and went further. Robert Tarone suggested that the women with abnormalities discovered when they entered the study should have been eliminated from it, and he called for a reanalysis of the data. Miller has always responded that there was no reason to eliminate those women because the numbers of women referred to the study surgeons were the same in both groups. As for Yaffe's concern that more women with advanced cancer were in the mammography group, the explanation is likely to do with where the abnormalities were diagnosed. A woman with a palpable lesion was likely assessed in a local centre. But if a woman had an impalpable lesion, detected only on a mammogram, she would have been assessed in a specialized centre, such as a teaching hospital, where standards of pathology, and thus the chance of finding involved lymph nodes, were higher.

Then Daniel Kopans made things really messy. Like Yaffe, he had questioned the randomization process in published articles. Now he accused Miller of scientific misconduct. Kopans claimed a radiology technician in Canada had personal knowledge of subversion. He officially complained to David Beatty, the head of the National Cancer Institute of Canada, and to Miller's boss, the dean of the Faculty of Medicine at the University of Toronto. This was serious stuff. It threatened Miller's reputation and possibly his job. Beatty spoke to Kopans and, after several attempts, made telephone contact with the technician in question. She told Beatty that on one social occasion she had made idle remarks on the subject, but not to Kopans. She declined to put any statements in writing. It turned out that she did not work at the centre where the alleged misconduct took place until two years after the randomization was complete.

Beatty thought the allegations were damning enough to call for an outside investigation that would report publicly. At great expense, the National Cancer Institute of Canada hired two scientists to conduct a review of the randomization. One was John Bailar, the epidemiologist who was at the NCI when controversies erupted over the Breast Cancer Detection Demonstration Project. He was now at McGill University in Montreal. The other was Brian MacMahon, an epidemiologist at the Harvard School of Public Health. At Bailar and MacMahon's request,

Beatty also hired document specialists from the firm KPMG. KPMG investigators examined the allocation lists for any evidence of alteration or substitution of names, one of the ways the randomization could be compromised. They inspected a total of 30,182 records.

Bailar and MacMahon published their review in the *Canadian Medical Association Journal* in 1997. They completely exonerated Miller. The investigation found no evidence of any subversion — only some clerical errors. But Yaffe and Kopans have never let it go. Twenty years later, Kopans rehashed at length everything he'd said many times before about the randomization in the journal *Breast Cancer Research and Treatment*. Even when something is not true, repeating it widely has a way of turning it into conventional wisdom that defies refutation.

The rift between Martin Yaffe and Anthony Miller epitomizes the polarization of mammography politics. Yaffe continues to argue strongly that women in their forties should have annual mammograms, even though none of the trials has shown that this would save lives. He continues to insist that the Canadian study is a flawed outlier. He offers his opinions frequently in letters to journals and to news media, championing breast screening and challenging those who don't. The deferential young physicist who knew little about cancer when he became part of the study is today a confident cancer crusader presiding over a prestigious research lab. Even though much of his work in digital mammography has been aimed at better diagnosis and treatment and screening is not his main focus, he promotes enhanced technology to help find breast cancer even earlier. His unshakeable belief in early detection is sincere. It's been a career pursuit.

But where does belief meet science? By the time Miller and Baines first published, belief was already a driving force in a fierce debate where the science that countered it was denigrated as faulty and dismissed. From the perspective of the believers, the Canadian study got the wrong answer. The only way they could explain it was to think there must have been a mistake, in spite of forensic investigation that proved otherwise. The mammogram wars, already bitter, were about to get even uglier.

Seven BRUTAL POLITICS

The room was tense with anticipation. The biggest names in mammography had been summoned to a Holiday Inn in Bethesda, Maryland, to submit and defend their latest breast-screening research. The shock of the controversial Canadian study's finding of no mortality benefit from routine mammograms was causing tremors in the United States, and the NCI could not ignore the developing intense, angry debate. The institute had been recommending annual mammograms for women starting at age forty. What if it was wrong? In late February 1993, just three months after the Canadian research made headlines around the globe, the NCI, looking for some guidance, called a meeting of international breast screening experts.

Sharon Batt felt the electricity the moment she entered the room. A shudder of excitement, like a collective frisson, signalled the importance of the event. She was a Canadian journalist doing a story for the CBC, and she took her place at the right along with the other journalists, among them Gina Kolata from the *New York Times* and Christine Russell from the *Washington Post*. Several television crews were there too. Although Batt was on assignment with a radio documentary to do, she had a deep, personal interest in the meeting. Five years earlier, a diagnosis of breast cancer at age forty-three turned her life upside down. Never having had a mammogram, she discovered the lump while soaping herself in the shower. The lump, in fact, didn't show up on the x-ray she subsequently had and was declared cancer only after a biopsy. She had a small tumour and some lymph nodes removed and then endured months of chemotherapy and six weeks of radiation. While she was going through all of that, she read one of Rose Kushner's books and, taking her cue, questioned her doctors at every step. A former editor of the Canadian consumer magazine *Protect Yourself,* Batt was now working on a book about the politics of breast cancer, in search of answers to questions she herself had as a confused patient. She was the co-founder and director of Breast Cancer Action Montreal, an advocacy group demanding better information and more respect from doctors, as well as a voice in policy decisions around treatment and prevention. Batt was an activist with a feminist, political perspective. For too long, she thought, others had spoken on patients' behalf.

Batt learned about the mammography screening controversy only after her diagnosis and treatment. But although she was aware of the dispute, she didn't expect what she was about to witness in Bethesda. She counted about 150 people in the low-ceilinged conference room, typically bland in beige and brown, with the exception of a bright yellow modern art piece hanging at the front. The mood was intense. Batt quickly discerned a distinct divide between the epidemiologists — the "public health people" — on one side and the radiologists on the other. Looking back more than thirty years later, she still sounds a little surprised by what unfolded. "I don't think I had ever witnessed that kind of vigorous debate," she says.

The goal of the two-day International Workshop on Screening for Breast Cancer was to review the current data from all the screening trials. In addition to the Canadian trial, there were four in Sweden, one in Scotland, and the earlier one in the United States, the New York HIP study. The trial leaders were invited to present their findings to a five-member scientific review panel. At the end of the second day, the reviewers would summarize the evidence and in the following month provide a report to the President's Cancer Panel, an advisory agency established in 1971 by the National Cancer Act. Getting all of the trial leaders together in the same room was enough to make this meeting historic. But the fireworks had yet to begin. This event would illustrate just how polarized the debate over screening had become and foreshadow what would happen through the remainder of the 1990s.

An honour roll of luminaries comprised the scientific panel: William Black, professor of radiology at Dartmouth-Hitchcock Medical Center in New Hampshire; Barbara Rimer, a professor at Duke University who later become dean of the Gillings School of Global Public Health at the University of North Carolina; Sam Shapiro, from the Johns Hopkins School of Hygiene and Public Health and a leader of the HIP study as well as a consultant on the Canadian study; and Russell Harris, an epidemiologist and internist from the University of North Carolina. Shapiro was now in his eighties; the others, much younger, remain, to this day, important voices on the issue of cancer screening. Suzanne Fletcher, co-editor of the *Annals of Internal Medicine*, chaired the panel.

She had excellent credentials for the job. Breast screening was not something Fletcher had even heard about when she entered medical school in 1962. Only in her second year, the year the HIP study began, did the subject come up. But cancer screening grew to be one of her major interests as she and her husband, Robert Fletcher, became fore-runners in the emerging field of clinical epidemiology. Up to then, the science of epidemiology was the study of patterns of disease and epidemics in large groups of people. Clinical epidemiologists measure how specific medical practices affect population health. They look at the effects of treatments, for example, or at preventive health measures and screening. What is the impact, say, of blood pressure monitoring on the incidence of cardiovascular disease or the overall effect on mortality when you introduce population-wide PSA tests for prostate cancer? This work became the focus of the Fletchers' careers, and together they wrote the first clinical epidemiology textbook. But first they headed to Montreal.

In the 1970s, the medical school at McGill University recruited them to teach the new epidemiology to its young doctors. They worked at McGill for five years, just at the time the new Canadian Task Force on the Periodic Health Examination got under way. The task force was set up to write guidelines for doctors on a multitude of everyday prac-tices, from cholesterol testing to Pap tests, based on the best evidence available. Suzanne Fletcher was a task force member from 1976 to 1979 and helped develop Canada's first national breast-screening guidelines.

When the United States adopted the Canadian model and established the US Preventive Services Task Force in 1984, Fletcher was one of the first to take part. Once again, she helped develop breast screening guidelines. Following Canada's lead, the American task force recommended mammography screening for women only after they turned fifty, but these recommendations were for doctors and not part of much public discussion. At the international meeting that February in 1993, however, the discussion was very much in the public. The meeting was open, media were there in force, and interested parties filled the chairs not occupied by experts and journalists. The place was packed.

Cornelia Baines was among the first speakers, there to present a review of the literature on breast self-examination. The more controversial matters were still to come, the most contentious being the questions around screening women under age fifty. Things heated up when Anthony Miller presented updated results from the Canadian study, the single trial among the seven under review uniquely designed to study women in their forties. When he said the results showed clearly that mammography screening did not save lives in that age group, Daniel Kopans launched an angry attack on behalf of the mammographers in the room. As usual, in an attempt to discredit the Canadian research, he argued that the mammograms were of poor quality. "Significant decisions are going to be made in this country on the basis of this study," Kopans said. "It is very important for us to know exactly what was done." He was vocal throughout the meeting, at one point dictating a statement he wanted included in the final report noting that no study had enough statistical power to conclude that mammograms were ineffective in women under fifty. Journalist Sharon Batt found his strident outbursts and ad hominem attacks on the Canadian researchers shocking.

But Miller had support from the other side, the public health people. New Zealand researcher Mark Elwood also riled the mammographers. He had attempted to pool the results of all the trials, which together included half a million women. This method of combining studies can sometimes offer a more telling picture than a single, smaller one. He reported that he could find no statistical benefit to screening women in their forties. Nancy Lee, a scientist with the Centers for Disease Control and Prevention, spoke up to say it was not possible to do perfect mammography in the field, and whatever faults the Canadian study might have had with its equipment, people, or training, its mammography was far better than in the average practice in the United States. "The Canadian study has probably more rigour than we have in our centres," she observed, and in that way was more "illustrative" than other research the radiologists touted. Batt found Miller's calm demeanour persuasive. "He was prepared. He knew he was going to be attacked. He had confidence in the study and the findings, and he just rolled with it," she recalls. "It was really quite impressive."

Suzanne Fletcher impressed Batt too. In her book *Patient No More*, she describes the fifty-two-year-old Fletcher as a tall, vibrant woman whose warm exuberance defused some of the tension. "I can't help admiring Fletcher's diplomacy," she writes. "She accentuates the positive and the field of consensus and understates the acrimony in the main area of disagreement." Today, Fletcher, now retired, still exudes kindness and tolerance for the views of others. She laughs a little at the mention of Daniel Kopans and recalls that he was indeed vocal in an aggressive way, but she says now, as she did then, that it's important to listen to what everyone has to say. Someone like Kopans, she notes, makes you think harder. It won't necessarily change your mind, but if you think harder, that's good.

At the end of the two-day workshop, Fletcher and the panel offered their assessment of both published and unpublished data. None of the screening trials showed a reduction in mortality as a result of screening women in their forties through the first seven years of follow-up. Some of the trials indicated a benefit after ten or more years of follow-up, but it was uncertain and, at best, marginal. Women in their forties experienced more harm from screening than women in their fifties, the panel concluded. More research was needed.

The second part of the Canadian study, the research on women aged fifty to fifty-nine, wasn't as relevant to the discussion as it differed from the other trials. Since all participants were given physical breast exams, there was no control group of unscreened women. That part of the trial was designed to test only whether adding mammography to a physical breast exam made any difference to death rates, so it couldn't be counted. The panel, analyzing all the other data, concluded that screening women over fifty reduced mortality by about a third. It was not a controversial finding.

What was highly contentious, however, was the question about women in their forties. The panel made no policy recommendations. Its job was only to summarize the data. But Kopans was not happy. He told the *New York Times* that every study was flawed and therefore could not satisfactorily answer the question about younger women. He had no choice but to rely on inference, he said, and he inferred that properly performed, good-quality mammograms will benefit women in their forties. Kopans said the same thing to a CBC television reporter: "Do we base our decisions on the fact we haven't studied the problem to get the absolute evidence?" he asked. "Or do we say that based on our experience over the years, the inferential data suggest we should be able to reduce the mortality and give women the benefit of the doubt." Yet his insistence that women should get a mammogram once a year hardly gave them the benefit of the doubt.

Women were beginning to realize that they were not getting the whole story. The morning after the workshop, Suzanne Fletcher picked up the *New York Times* and was surprised to see a report from Gina Kolata on the front page. "Studies Say Mammograms Fail to Help Many Women," read the headline, prominently placed at the top left. Fletcher was still at the hotel when someone from the NCI asked if she would meet with some "quite upset" representatives of breast cancer advocacy groups. She encountered a clutch of women frustrated and angry, not about the panel's conclusions, but at what they hadn't been told. Until then, they had no idea that screening women in their forties was surrounded with so much uncertainty. They resented that the scientific community was withholding information. They told Fletcher it was patronizing.

That's exactly how Cindy Pearson felt. She was a staff member of the National Women's Health Network, based in Washington, DC, and it was part of her job to monitor what took place at the workshop. It was eye opening, she remembers. "For us, it was like, holy cow, all these researchers know that it is not as effective for women in their forties as it is for older women, and no one is saying that to women." In the burgeoning feminism of the time, advocacy groups such as Pearson's and Sharon Batt's group in Montreal were demanding that women have a voice in their health care: in childbirth issues, in contraception, in breast cancer treatment. Inspired by *Our Bodies, Ourselves*, the bible of female health published by the Boston Women's Health Book Collective, women were insisting on a different relationship with their doctors. They no longer wanted to be patted on the head and told condescendingly what to do. And in their insistence on good care, they had fought for the right to have mammography screening without having to pay for it. But after the 1993 workshop, some groups, including the National Women's Health Network, began to back away from telling women to get screened. For Cindy Pearson, it was an epiphany. It was also a moment of awakening for Suzanne Fletcher. The women she met with were right to be angry.

Women weren't getting information about the limitations of screening. They were told only that screening saves lives, and sometimes the messaging was outright arrogant. These days an audience of women — and men — gasps when shown an American Cancer Society print ad from 1990 featuring a tight shot of a woman's face with the caption "If you haven't had a mammogram, you need more than your breasts examined." The ad urged women to begin annual screening at age thirty-five. Except for a brief period in the 1970s, the American Cancer Society had always promoted screening for women under fifty. It knew how to run campaigns and understood the impact of television. One powerful commercial borrowed from the iconic shower scene in the movie *Psycho*.

Eerie music portends danger as the camera peers through a set of French doors at a woman in a pink bathrobe. "A killer is loose," intones the male narrator. The camera follows the woman from behind, stalking her as she walks through a spacious living room furnished with luxurious Persian rugs and plush white furniture. Lamps create deep shadows on the wall. As she latches the door to the hallway, she pauses, head tilted as if she hears something. A close-up reveals that she is forty-something, pretty. White lace rims the collar of her robe, framing an intelligent, confident-looking face and dark curls in a ponytail. She turns back toward another room. The deep voice drones: "Regardless of age, race, income, family background, it strikes. Breast cancer is a killer." The music intensifies. Quick cuts speed up the action: robe tossed on a bed, bare foot stepping into the shower, a turn of the faucet. Then a wide shot, her silhouette through the glass shower door. The camera moves in. The killer is getting closer. The narration resumes: "Don't be a victim. Fight back. Mammography. Your most powerful weapon."

The TV ad is goosebump-creepy but effective. The American Cancer Society has come to the damsel's rescue.

Over at the NCI, these simplistic messages were causing growing unease. The institute had initially embraced screening for women in their forties when, in 1973, it joined forces with the American Cancer Society in the Breast Cancer Detection Demonstration Project, offering free screening in twenty-seven centres across the United States. Midway through the five-year project, the institute determined that healthy women under fifty should not be screened. In 1989, the NCI revised its policy again after accepting an invitation from the American College of Radiology to join a meeting of organizations interested in forming consistent recommendations on screening. It agreed that women aged forty to forty-nine should get a clinical breast exam every year and a screening mammogram every one to two years.

But now, with the publication of the Canadian study and the data gathered at the international workshop, the NCI had to reconsider. Director Samuel Broder was not comfortable with continuing to support a guideline advising screening for younger women. With Suzanne Fletcher's report in hand, he said publicly he couldn't see how anyone could claim mammography saves lives when there wasn't any statistical evidence to support it. He signalled a dramatic change in thinking and ignited a fierce political battle.

In September 1993, Broder proposed a revised guideline to his overseer, the National Cancer Advisory Board. The guideline would recommend that women aged forty to forty-nine should "discuss with a health professional the advisability of screening with mammography, taking into account family history of breast cancer and other risk factors." It would also recommend "annual clinical breast examination as a prudent practice for this age group." The advisory board refused to accept the change. Daniel Kopans, who had written letters to every board member, was delighted, but only briefly, because in December, the NCI swerved around the controversy with an alternative approach. Instead of a guideline, it issued what it called a summary of scientific fact. "Experts do not agree on the role of routine screening mammography for women ages forty to forty-nine," the summary stated. "To date, randomized clinical trials have not shown a statistically significant reduction in mortality for women under the age of fifty."

In arguments about health policy, cost is typically a factor in the politics. While the NCI was trying to revise its screening recommendations, President Bill Clinton and First Lady Hillary Clinton were in the midst of constructing a health-care plan. In their proposal, the plan would not pay for routine mammograms for women in their forties due to the evidence of no benefit. The average mammogram cost one hundred dollars. An estimated five million women under fifty had one each year, at a total cost of half-a-billion dollars. Forty-two states had laws forcing private insurers to pay for those mammograms. If the Clinton health plan resulted in changes to private insurance, not only would it cause financial hardship for some women who wanted mammograms regardless, but also the mammogram industry stood to lose a great deal of income. The NCI was under pressure from lobby groups and politicians. Early in 1994, Congress summoned Broder to a hearing to defend the institute's position. The NCI had created confusion by backing off from a clear guideline and offering instead a non-prescriptive summary of scientific fact. What were women, doctors, and insurance plans supposed to do with a statement that said experts don't agree? In the void the lack of direction left, the fight over screening women predictably continued.

Barnett Kramer was in the midst of that fight. He is currently director of cancer prevention at the NCI, but in 1993, he was deputy director and one of the organizers of the international workshop in Bethesda. An internal medicine and oncology specialist with expertise in screening issues, he was also the editor of the *Journal of the National Cancer Institute*. The community of experts who promote evidence-based medicine and who are concerned about overdiagnosis and overtreatment hail Kramer as mentor. At a recent conference in Quebec City, where he was the first keynote speaker, the chair introduced him as a "hero." A man of slight build and thin voice, who casually carries a backpack over his suit as he makes his way through a crowded meeting room, Kramer is the kind of person people find easy to talk to. He has unrivalled respect as a trailblazer in forward-thinking medicine but is unassuming and generous with his knowledge. Everyone calls him Barry.

The heat from the Canadian screening study had an impact in his office, not only because it was controversial. The NCI was already questioning whether it should have any part in setting guidelines, feeling that the job of a science agency is to convey scientific knowledge, not offer recommendations on behaviour to the public. Kramer was among those who wanted to get out of the business of guidelines and policy-making, especially after the fuss over mammography. He also had ethical concerns about how guidelines were made. "It wouldn't have met the standards that are currently considered the best methods for developing a guideline," he says about the breast-screening recommendation. People chosen to be part of a consensus panel weren't vetted for conflicts of interest. They represented specialty societies that often had pre-established strong positions, their minds made up before they became part of the panel.

In the context of the breast-screening debate, Kramer's point is an important one. Radiologists invented breast screening; they were considered the experts. For a long time, they owned the screening issue. But who should decide public policy? Should those who stand to gain financially get to make the rules or even take part in the rule making? The US Preventive Services Task Force, the body that sets national guidelines today, was establishing a more formal approach, where analytical skills and understanding of research methodology took precedence over specialty expertise. Eventually, the NCI would cede all of its guidelines to that agency, but not before another big flare-up in the mammography debate.

In 1997, Kramer watched it all happen. The NCI decided it was time to try to end the lingering confusion over screening women in their forties. Richard Klausner, the new director, was a physician and a biomedical research scientist. He came to the job envisioning a more scientific approach to the detection and treatment of cancer than the experimental approach of the past. For instance, he says, chemotherapy was developed through trying out different combinations of drugs to see what could work. It was trial and error, stabbing in the dark. He wanted the NCI to lead the global cancer community into more methodical approaches.

When Klausner heard about new data on mammography coming out of a meeting in Falun, Sweden, in 1996, he thought if there was new evidence, the NCI's 1993 summary-of-fact statement should be revisited. The Swedish data were not yet published or peer reviewed, but they were positive for screening. Hearing from an NCI staffer who attended the Falun meeting that the data could change the game, Klausner saw a chance to finally resolve the debate about screening women in their forties. He proposed an NIH consensus conference, confident that under formal rules and with an unbiased panel, the benefits and risks of screening could be discussed in a neutral setting.

Once again, Kramer served on the planning committee, the size of which was an indication of the size and importance of the conference. It had thirty-two members, most of them scientists from the NIH and academics from medical colleges. Anthony Miller was on the committee, as well as László Tabár, the Swedish Two-County trial researcher.

Daniel Kopans, who was anything but neutral, was not involved at first. He told *Science* magazine the NCI intended to stack the deck against screening, and he had to lobby his way into the planning meetings. Miller wasn't the only person on the committee who had suffered attacks from Kopans. Kramer also had been a target. Kopans disagreed with the *Journal of the National Cancer Institute*'s editorial choices and wrote not only to Kramer's bosses but also to politicians and the media to complain. That kind of pushy insistence got Kopans a seat at the planning committee.

The second NIH consensus development conference on breast screening, this time focusing solely on women in their forties, took place twenty years after the first, from January 21 to 23, 1997, in the Natcher Auditorium on the NIH campus in Bethesda. The venue was modern, only three years old, but constructed like an Italian opera house. Three balconies line up horizontally at the back of a narrow hall, and although it can hold a thousand delegates, the auditorium can feel close. This conference was jammed; even the balconies were full. In preparation, the thirteen-member panel had been given an extensive reading list. Now it had three days to develop consensus guidelines, and the schedule was precise. The panel would spend the first day and a half hearing from a roster of invited speakers before retiring to a separate meeting room, as if sequestered, to deliberate. Its task was to answer a series of questions. Did screening women in their forties reduce mortality, and how large was the benefit? What were the risks? Were there other benefits? What were the directions for future research? On the third and final morning of the conference, the panel chair would present a draft statement to the conference, there would be discussion and questions from the audience, and then the panel would retreat once more to consider any changes. A press conference would follow in the afternoon. Never was a meeting better intentioned or more meticulously planned. Yet it ended in disaster. "It was just bedlam," Kramer says. Suzanne Fletcher, chair of the 1993 panel and a speaker at this much larger conference, compared it to the scene in *Alice in Wonderland* where the queen declares, "Sentence first, verdict afterwards," before shouting, "Off with her head!" Cornelia Baines was also a speaker and shudders at the memory of "an appalling experience."

The meeting was raucous from the beginning. During the first day and a half of presentations, says Kramer, "it was already clear that feelings were running high." A presentation from New Zealand researcher Brian Cox triggered a lot of anger and debate. Cox, a public health physician, had done a meta-analysis, an aggregation of data from a number of clinical trials. He added the mortality statistics from the different breast-screening trials and estimated little or no benefit from screening women in their forties. He might as well have waved a red cape at the screening proponents in the audience. From Sweden, another meta-analysis offered results positive for screening. Meta-analyses are tricky. If the individual trials aren't exactly the same, adding up the results can be misleading, even wrong. But they played a big role at this conference, fuelling the debate.

The screening advocates in the crowd began to put forward data that had been neither published nor reviewed. Kramer recalls that they were busy making phone calls and doing their own hasty analyses. "They would just do quick and dirty meta-analyses on the fly, hour by hour, during the course of that day and a half." They spoke from the floor during discussion periods. "The poor panel," says Kramer, had to deal with to-and-fro, see-sawing arguments about material they had never seen. "That added to the free-for-all aspect."

The panel sat facing the audience at a long table on the stage, and speakers came up to a podium, also on the stage. Donald Berry, a statistician at Duke University and vice-chair of the panel, wasn't prepared for the fervour he witnessed as he looked out at the crowd. A particularly noisy moment occurred when one of the pro-screening statisticians in the audience jumped up from the floor to proclaim at the microphone that he now had statistical significance. A chorus of cheers went up. "It was like a revival meeting," chuckles Berry, "with hallelujahs." Statistical significance is a benchmark scientists rely on to know that an effect they observe is highly likely to be real and not just due to random chance. If you take a pill and feel better, is it truly because of the pill, or is it just a coincidence? It's why drugs are measured against placebos to test whether they work. Often two things happening at the same time give the appearance of cause and effect when that's not the case. We know, for instance, that the rooster does not make the sun come up. Sometimes, however, statisticians manipulate numbers in order to find a statistically significant result, for example, in a particular subsection of people in a study. It may be irrelevant to the overall picture and entirely misleading. That's what the statistician at the podium did, says Berry, but the crowd loved it. He could tell by the intensity of the hallelujahs that the audience was largely a homogeneous group of radiologists. He was beginning to understand the politics.

Day two was a marathon for the panellists. Proceedings began at eight a.m., and then the panel settled down after lunch to hash out a consensus. They didn't wrap up until three a.m. the next morning. Leon Gordis, an epidemiologist from Johns Hopkins University, an eminent scientist, and the panel's chair, earned much respect for his ability to manage the discussion and keep the atmosphere as cordial as it could be among a group of bleary-eyed people under pressure to agree. The disparate bunch included two professors of radiology, two obstetrician-gynecologists, two patient advocates, and a professor of geriatrics plus statisticians and epidemiologists. Later, it would come out that they did not reach a consensus, but that's not how the chair and the panel presented it the next day.

A draft statement was available for conference participants to read early on the morning of day three, before things got under way. That's when bedlam really erupted. The way things had been going, with so much emotion in the auditorium, many expected that the panel would find in favour of screening. The meeting was in for a surprise. The panel concluded that the evidence did not warrant a recommendation for screening all women in their forties. If screening saved any lives at all, it might save, at best, ten out of ten thousand screened every year for ten years. But over the decade, 30 percent may have false positive results or treatment for a cancer that would never cause any problems. A woman should make her own decision after being given the best possible information about the benefits and risks. The panel advocated for educational material to be developed for women, and for their doctors, to arm them with the best possible information about benefits and risks before making their own decisions. For women who chose mammography, the group said, insurance plans should cover the cost. It wasn't a hardline conclusion. The panel didn't exactly say no to mammography but simply that it lacked the data to support saying yes. The nuance was lost in the ensuing melee.

The room was rumbling when the panellists entered that morning. The moment Leon Gordis began to read the consensus statement, people rushed to the microphones. Eyes filled with tears. An angry Kopans denounced the panel's report as fraudulent. It was "tantamount to a death sentence for thousands of women," charged Michael Linver, a radiologist from New Mexico. "I grieve for them." One screening proponent got so worked up he reportedly shoved a member of NCI staff, saying the findings were unacceptable. Reporters spotted Richard Klausner, the NCI's director, rushing out to the hallway and went after him. The next day, the *New York Times* quoted him saying he was "shocked" by the panel's decision. He explained days later in a radio interview that the acrimony in the room is what shocked him, not the panel's conclusions.

One of the oddest moments of the entire meeting occurred at the press conference. Klausner was not supposed to be part of it, but when a journalist wanted to ask him a question, he walked up from the audience to the podium and in doing so essentially took over. Many in the room were stunned when he contradicted the panel with his personal opinion on the mortality benefit from screening. "My own evaluation of the data is that the data supporting the benefit of initiating screening in the forties is stronger than it had been," he said. The National Cancer Advisory Board, he said, would discuss the conference at its next meeting. As Klausner exited, the media followed him with more questions, and the press conference ended with the panel abandoned on stage, perplexed. Klausner had undermined the scientists he had brought together for a meeting he created. The audience cheered him.

Leon Gordis and the panel were bewildered. They had spent weeks reading more than a hundred scientific papers and hundreds more abstracts and had come to the consensus conference wanting to achieve a meaningful outcome. They had been up half the night reviewing what all of the speakers had said, listening carefully to what each of the other panellists had to say. Their deliberations were thoughtful, patient, and collegial — intense but not contentious. The hostility that greeted them the next morning, to be told that the death of women would be on their heads, was devastating. Gordis was furious at how Klausner had dismissed the panel's consensus statement and hijacked the press conference.

Connie Rufenbarger found it emotional and exhausting. A patient advocate from Indiana, Rufenbarger is a volunteer who continues to serve on the executive of the group she was working with at the time of the consensus conference, the Catherine Peachey Fund. She had been unusually young, only thirty-four, when she learned she had breast cancer in 1981. Surgery was the only option as there were no other treatments offered then, neither chemotherapy nor radiation. Rufenbarger had a full mastectomy of one breast. At the time, she recalls, breasts and breast cancer were such shameful subjects to discuss in public that it was difficult to even utter the words. In silent ignorance, Rufenbarger didn't know enough to be afraid. Besides, she had children to raise. But watching a friend die of the disease turned her into an activist, and since then she has helped countless women get through the ordeal and grieved for many who did not. As someone who had set up mammography screening clinics, she arrived at the consensus conference wanting to recommend screening for women in their forties. She told the angry throng no one wanted to make that recommendation more than she did. But she couldn't. The evidence to support it did not exist. Rufenbarger says today, "I knew in my heart there was only one thing I could do." But it was difficult, and when it was over, it was like being in recovery, not made any easier by some passionate letters and phone calls from people who wanted to tell her she was wrong.

Washington politicians reacted immediately. Within days, the Senate voted ninety-eight to zero for a resolution calling for the National Cancer Advisory Board to recommend screening women in their forties. Senator Arlen Specter summoned Klausner, Gordis, and other consensus panel members to testify before Congress. Specter chaired a committee that dealt with appropriations for the department responsible for the NIH and the NCI. His wife had breast cancer, so he had a special interest in screening, and he was livid. He called Klausner on the phone and threatened not only to have his job but also to cancel the NCI's budget. The senator was insistent that screening benefited women in their forties, and he wanted the NCI to declare a clear policy to deal with the confusion resulting from the consensus conference. He held three special congressional hearings over the next month. Klausner appeared at the first one, on February 5, just two weeks after the consensus conference fiasco, to assure senators that the mammography question remained open and that the NCI would abide by guidance from the National Cancer Advisory Board.

Another powerful voice in the mammography debate emerged at those hearings. Fran Visco was the president of the National Breast Cancer Coalition, an organization she had helped establish in 1991 to lobby politically for more research into breast cancer prevention and treatment. Visco was a lawyer in Philadelphia who in 1987 was diagnosed with breast cancer at the age of thirty-nine. She knew nothing about the disease. Having no family history, she didn't think she needed to pay much attention. But her gynecologist recommended a screening mammogram. It revealed that not only did she have a lump, but the cancer had spread to her lymph nodes. She needed a lumpectomy, radiation, and chemotherapy for a type of cancer that had a poorer prognosis than some other breast cancers. She was scared for her life, but what also troubled her was that the medical profession had few answers about why some people get breast cancer, why some survive whereas others don't, and why such toxic treatments were necessary. Visco abandoned the law in favour of activism after she became the National Breast Cancer Coalition's first president.

She knew Senator Specter as he, too, was from Philadelphia, and he invited her to appear twice at his hearings. But she was no fan of screening. The science had convinced her that screening did not save lives, and she wanted breast cancer resources spent elsewhere. She argued that women weren't getting the facts. "We all want it to be simple," she told the hearing. "We want mammography to work in all women. It doesn't. We want to reduce breast cancer to a sound bite. It cannot be. We cannot continue to sell women false hope simply because we do not want them to be confused."

The National Cancer Advisory Board, called to action by Klausner, was also confronting political reality. Klausner met with members of the board several times. He needed them to contradict the consensus panel's conclusions. Kay Dickersin, an epidemiologist at the University of Maryland School of Medicine, remembers that the board tried to get Klausner to understand the science. Dickersin was a breast cancer survivor who'd had a double mastectomy a decade earlier, at age thirty-four, and was active in the National Breast Cancer Coalition. Wearing two hats, scientist and consumer advocate, she knew the consensus panel was right. Still, the threat of the NCI losing its funding was also real. The advisory board would have to vote, and she struggled with her conscience. Two months after the consensus meeting, the advisory board recommended that the NCI adopt a guideline advising women aged forty to forty-nine to have screening mammograms every one to two years. The board had eighteen members. Dickersin cast the one dissenting vote.

Arlen Specter got what he wanted. The NCI reversed its 1993 position. The institute issued a statement jointly with the American Cancer Society saying the two groups agreed that screening women in their forties is "beneficial and supportable with current scientific evidence." Within hours, President Clinton, in a White House press briefing, applauded the NCI for providing "consistent guidance" and called upon third-party insurers to cover screening costs. (By this time, Clinton had been forced to give up his health plan, which would not have paid for mammograms for women under fifty. But women's issues were still part of his platform, and he was getting a clear message from Congress.) The "consistent" message from the NCI would not change again for more than a decade. Brutal politics would once more play out when, in 2009, the US Preventive Services Task Force wrote a guideline suggesting that the evidence for screening younger women was insufficient. But for now, the screening supporters had won the mammogram wars.

As was eventually made clear, when details from the consensus conference were published in the *Journal of the National Cancer Institute* several months later, there had not been a true consensus. Two panel members who did not go along with the initial recommendation wrote a minority report. They thought the evidence was good enough to justify a policy of screening women in their forties. Told they would be able to write a minority report, they agreed to conform to the majority in the final statement. A third panellist who also disagreed with the majority resigned, and her name appears in neither the majority nor the minority report.

For Barry Kramer, the consensus conference and the aftermath were sobering. "I had never been in a scientific conference where there was so much anger," he sighs. He continued to work at getting the NCI out of the guideline business, finally succeeding just a few years ago. Richard Klausner left the institute in 2001, after only six years. He loved his job, he said when he announced his resignation, but he wanted to be closer to research. Not long after, he headed west to become executive director for global health at the Bill & Melinda Gates Foundation for three years. From there he went into the biotechnology industry.

Reflecting on his years at the NCI, Klausner confesses that the front-page article in the *New York Times*, the one that quoted him saying the consensus conference decision was "shocking," was the lowest point during his time as director. He blames himself for the reaction to his comment at the press conference, where he appeared to undermine the consensus panel. That was not his intention. He was trying to reassure everyone "that the NCI and I were listening to all voices." Just because, looking at the data, a group of independent people went one way didn't mean there weren't data in support of another position. The real mistake on his part, he thinks, was in not understanding how he was going to be interpreted, "not having been more aware of the parsing of words." Twenty years later, Klausner thinks we've come close to the conference consensus. He claims that he wasn't a mammography advocate at the time and is even less so now. The ongoing debate, he says, represents "the simple fact that it's really a lousy screening method compared to the methods we wish we had."

When journalist Sharon Batt went to the first conference in 1993, she wanted to make sense of the whole thing. There was this idea that if you just had perfect, up-to-date equipment, mammography would work. It seemed to her, even then, that wasn't the whole story. "Really, it's a flawed technology. It's too expensive for what it does, gives you too many false positives, too many false negatives. It's something that's been latched on to because people were concerned about breast cancer." Batt didn't stick with breast cancer activism. She left Montreal for an academic position in women's studies at Mount Saint Vincent University in Nova Scotia in 1999. She had completed a master's degree in sociology before going into journalism, and this opportunity was the beginning of a new career in academia. She studied for a PhD at Dalhousie University in Halifax and now teaches bioethics. She recently published a second book investigating the relationship between patient advocates and the pharmaceutical industry.

Connie Rufenbarger had a second bout of cancer in her healthy breast, when she was fifty-two, two years after the consensus conference. The tumour was tiny, but she opted for a mastectomy, not wanting to go through months of treatment. She hasn't changed her mind about the consensus panel finding the evidence insufficient to warrant screening in women under fifty.

Fran Visco continues to serve as the president of the National Breast Cancer Coalition and also has not changed her mind. The coalition's position is that screening at any age results in a modest mortality benefit that is outweighed by its cost and its harms. But the marketing of early detection has created what she calls a "ridiculous myth" that mammography screening is a panacea, "completely ignoring the fact we're intervening in a healthy population." And if you are intervening in a healthy population, she says, "you better be careful that you're doing much more good than harm." Those views have earned her and the coalition plenty of animosity. "It's out of control," Visco sighs. "The hatred and the vehemence with which people react when anyone questions mammography is mind boggling."

Cornelia Baines describes her feelings about the consensus debacle as "slightly surprised and slightly indignant" because by then she was becoming accustomed to the breast-screening politics and had come to "generalize the experience to what happens in the rest of the world." She adds with sadness in her voice, "We believe the stories that people in power choose to tell us." When the belief that mammography saves lives is profoundly prevalent, trying to write the scientific truth in academic journals doesn't get you anywhere, she believes now. "Yes, we convince people who intelligently evaluate evidence, but no, we do not influence the people with conflicts of interest, and we do not influence the people who have been brainwashed to be afraid of breast cancer and have been brainwashed to believe that mammography saves lives." By the end of the 1990s, it was clear that the mammography screening debate was not really a debate about science. It was about belief. The Canadian study was maligned not for its technical failures but because it said something many people did not want to hear.

Eight   VINDICATION

A few days after her seventy-sixth birthday, Penny Gerrie bought a new bicycle. Her old no-gear coaster bike had served her well for many years, but it was heavy, and she was finding it increasingly difficult to lift it up the front steps and into the foyer of the house where she rents an apartment. Use of her sister's seven-speed for a while convinced her of the value of gears when navigating hills. So that's what she chose: a seven-speed in a low-key muted bronze, a colour she hoped would not attract the attention of thieves. Neither fancy nor fussy, the bike is a practical mode of transportation for someone who doesn't own a car.

Gerrie lives in Toronto and regularly cycles long distances from one end of the city to the other. Long before the city developed its current network of bike lanes, she decided that cycling was more convenient than public transit. She also enjoys the exercise. For the same reasons, she has always walked a lot, and a seven-kilometre route was once a three-times-a-week routine. On a nice day, she'd meet a friend for lunch downtown, an hour away on foot, and walk another hour back. She's thin and fit, with a confident posture. Her elegant short hair, good bones, and stylish dress complete a striking picture that disguises her age by at least a decade. She could be a fashion model.

Health conscious but not obsessive about it, Gerrie is the kind of person who sees a doctor only when she needs to. In the summer of 2016, she began to experience some worrying pain in her hips and knees on her long walks. The mobility she took for granted seemed to be slipping away, and wanting to do something about it, or at least find out what was going on, she made an appointment. Her doctor decided to order x-rays. When a look at Gerrie's chart revealed that she hadn't had any of the usual screening tests for at least five years, she also suggested a colonoscopy, a bone density test, and a mammogram. Gerrie dutifully consented. At this point, she was a healthy seventy-five-year-old seeking pain relief. She'd soon find herself spiralling down a medical rabbit hole.

The x-rays revealed some minor arthritis in her right hip for which her doctor advised physiotherapy. It was a relief that the diagnosis wasn't serious and that preventing pain was possible. That done, she went for the other tests, all arranged in the same week in the middle of October. A few days after the mammogram, the breast-screening clinic called to request that she come in again for additional mammography of the right breast. Like many women, Gerrie had been called back for a second mammogram once before. It happens. Sometimes the images aren't quite clear enough. *No big deal*, she thought. But the woman on the phone insisted that she get it done at the earliest possible date. She also told her to prepare to be there a few hours, in case she needed a biopsy. Gerrie was more annoyed than worried. She'd have to miss a special movie showing she'd been looking forward to.

She returned to the clinic on October 31, just two weeks after the first mammogram. The new images confirmed a small lump, a tiny mass not big enough to feel. She was ushered to another room for a core needle biopsy. Before proceeding, the doctor studied the original mammograms of both breasts, as well as the new ones of the right, and his eye caught something suspicious, unnoticed before, in the left breast. He decided to biopsy that too. In her typically practical approach to things, Gerrie appreciated the convenience of having both biopsies done at once. The procedure was painless, with no after-effects. She went home to await the results.

Her family physician gave her the news on the phone. It shouldn't have happened that way, but an emergency in the doctor's family meant that an office visit could not be immediately arranged. Both lumps were cancer, the doctor told her, but they were very small, and she would likely not need more than simple lumpectomies. Gerrie's first meeting with her surgeon, on November 21, was also reassuring. She would have the lumpectomies in just two weeks. She doesn't remember being afraid. Her elder sister had been diagnosed with breast cancer at the same age, five years earlier, and always said it was a piece of cake. Gerrie quipped in an email that she was concerned only about not being able to lift more than ten pounds for the first two weeks after the surgery. She also griped about the "stupid" questionnaires at every stop, always repeating the same questions. "I swear I gave them four different dates for the start of menstruation," she said. "I just couldn't remember." She was grateful to the radiologist who found the lump in the second breast, thinking if he hadn't been so thorough, she'd be going through all of this again in a few years.

On December 7, less than eight weeks from the first mammogram, she was in the operating room. The rapid pace at which one appointment led to the next and then to the next didn't leave much time to think about anything except stocking the fridge and getting organized. Gerrie had begun physiotherapy for her hip, but she let that slide in the whirlwind the diagnosis of breast cancer created. She lives alone but is fiercely self-sufficient, and she told friends not to worry, that a close neighbour would take her home from hospital and be on call for anything she needed. Everything was under control.

She glided smoothly through recovery without much pain — only some discomfort from bruising and swelling and irritation at having to sleep in a bra. The pathology report indicated two tiny tumours, the one in the right breast only six millimetres in diameter and the one in the left only five millimetres. No lymph nodes were involved. Gerrie had a low-grade stage-one cancer, classified as ER-positive, a kind that is less aggressive than others. This was all good news, but she didn't yet know what follow-up treatment she would need. Her file was now in the hands of an oncologist.

She waited three more weeks. The day she met the oncologist was one of those dreary, cloudy days when you don't know whether to expect rain, snow, or both. It's weather that chills to the bone. Such an ominous, oppressive hovering in the air makes it hard to have an optimistic outlook. But Gerrie was in for a surprise. The oncologist, a specialist in chemotherapy and drug treatments, was frank in a way she didn't expect. Did she know about overdiagnosis? And overtreatment? He explained that overdiagnosis of breast cancer happens to a lot of older women. If she had never had a mammogram, she would likely have lived another ten or twenty years without even knowing she had tumours in her breasts. They might never have caused any problems. Go home, he prescribed, and celebrate a Happy New Year. He wasn't going to advise any further treatment. *Wow,* she thought, *he just told me that it was all unnecessary.*

She still had to see a radiation specialist. Even though she wouldn't need drug or chemotherapy, she thought radiation might be recommended. That didn't happen either. The specialist told her that without treatment, the chance of the cancer recurring within ten years was about 15 percent. So how would she feel about risking another lumpectomy instead of undergoing any radiation? he asked. She was fine with that. He asked her to think about the radiation, but he was not at all insistent on it. It reaffirmed what she was already thinking, that all she had been through in the last few months was pointless.

Gerrie was aware of some of the issues around mammography screening, but she followed her family doctor's advice because, as she says, "You just do." She wishes now that the kindly oncologist had been the first doctor she'd seen in her breast cancer journey. But overdiagnosis is complicated. It's easy to understand that mammograms sometimes give false positive results, meaning that whatever is detected on the image turns out to be innocent when biopsied. Women are also warned that mammograms can miss cancers. It's never been a perfect test. Overdiagnosis, however, refers to the phenomenon where the cancer is real yet indolent, and the consequence is unnecessary surgery followed by unnecessary chemotherapy or radiation. The conundrum is that it's currently not possible to know which cancers will remain indolent. Once they're detected, ignoring them is not an option. Gerrie's oncologist could not have told her for certain, and she will never know, what would have happened if no one had squeezed her breasts into a mammography machine.

Three months after the lumpectomies, Gerrie was still feeling some numbness under her right arm, and she was unhappy about being lopsided, with one breast smaller than the other. Corrective surgery was a possibility, but she didn't even want to think about another operation. The thing that bothered her most was that she had put aside the issues with her hips and knees. The pain had become much more severe in the last few months, and when she was done with breast cancer, she saw a rheumatologist and had more x-rays. This time, the diagnosis was severe arthritis in the right hip and moderate arthritis in the left. She wonders if she would be in this "pickle," as she calls it, if the breast cancer hadn't distracted her from worrying about her joints. Adding to her frustration, arranging follow-up on the arthritis diagnosis was slow in comparison with the speed with which she was ushered through the cancer protocol. It would take nearly a year before she finally had hip surgery.

Penny Gerrie was seventy-five when her doctor sent her for a routine mammogram. Most public breast screening programs stop inviting women at age seventy, and none extend the routine screening age beyond age seventy-four. The fact that her sister had breast cancer was no doubt a consideration in the family doctor's mind, and it was in Gerrie's too. Family history is often assumed to be a major risk factor, although research shows that in older women, it is far less significant than either dense breasts or obesity. But Gerrie never considered the risk of overdiagnosis and potential overtreatment until she saw the oncologist.

Hers was the kind of scenario that makes Peter Gøtzsche angry. He's been researching and writing about overdiagnosis and the harm that can result for many years and can take credit for being the person who did the most to try to get the world to understand the magnitude of the problem. Others had talked about this worrisome side effect of mammography screening, but it was his work at the Nordic Cochrane Centre in Denmark that brought it to the foreground. In the beginning, however, his research was unpopular and suppressed, and he was attacked. It was therefore with some trepidation that he agreed to speak to a conference of breast cancer activists in Washington, DC, on a Sunday morning in May 2001. Gøtzsche stood at the podium with an eye on the exit doors. He had arrived early and scoped them out before he was scheduled to speak so that he could escape if "hundreds of women started to throw tomatoes and eggs" at him. It was unlikely that the audience would hurl anything more than a few questions his way, but he was about to tell a crowd of cancer survivors that mammography screening doesn't work. He had no idea how they would react.

The National Breast Cancer Coalition had invited him to speak at its annual meeting because of a paper he had written for the *Lancet*. It was a new analysis of the randomized breast screening trials that was stirring up a whole new round of fighting in the bitter mammogram wars and getting a lot of attention from patient groups such as the one he was addressing today. Seven hundred women from across the United States were gathered in the grand ballroom of the JW Marriott Hotel on Pennsylvania Avenue, just steps from the White House. Gøtzsche was on a panel with Anthony Miller and the radiologist Stephen Feig titled "Putting the Evidence into Breast Cancer Care — Challenges and Controversies for the Future."

He had suffered repeated condemnation for his message about screening; he had learned to anticipate hostility. This time was different. When he concluded his talk, a smile of surprise came across his face as he realized that the majority of the women in the audience were standing up to applaud. "I could have cried," Gøtzsche wrote many years later. "It was one of the most moving moments of my career." He was humbled that "these brave women who fought so hard against their breast cancer" welcomed what he had to say.

As improbable as eggs and tomatoes would be at such an event, it's also hard to imagine that this tough-minded scientist would be intimidated. His mission is to find the truth in other scientists' work. He began his career as a biologist in Denmark and was working in clinical research at the Swedish pharmaceutical company Astra in the

1970s when he decided to go into medicine. While doing research on insulin, he stumbled upon some conflict-of-interest issues, and that, plus a love of mathematics, led him to study bias in clinical research. In addition to directing the Nordic Cochrane Centre, he is a professor of clinical research design at the University of Copenhagen.

The Nordic Cochrane Centre is part of a global network of researchers, health professionals, and patients dedicated to independent, evidence-based reviews of clinical trials. The network, originally known as the Cochrane Collaboration and now simply Cochrane, is a non-profit organization widely praised for the quality of its impartial analyses of existing studies to assess the effectiveness of drugs and other medical interventions. Cochrane takes no money from the pharmaceutical industry or any other commercial source. Its reviews are a valuable, trusted source for individual doctors making treatment decisions and for policy-makers. The organization is named for Archie Cochrane, a Scottish physician concerned about the lack of science behind much of what doctors practised who advocated rigorous and well-designed studies to know whether a treatment or procedure worked. His 1972 book, *Effectiveness & Efficiency: Random Reflections on Health Services*, hugely influenced medicine and epidemiological research. Like David Sackett, who promoted similar ideas at McMaster University in Canada, Cochrane is considered a father of evidence-based medicine. He died in 1988, but one of his adherents carried on his work. Iain Chalmers was director of the National Perinatal Epidemiology Unit at Oxford University for many years and developed a database where physicians could consult reviews of trials involving care in pregnancy and childbirth. The National Health Service decided to do the same for other areas of health care and appointed Chalmers as the first director of the UK Cochrane Centre in 1992. A year later, Chalmers organized an international meeting to create the Cochrane Collaboration. Today, the organization has fourteen centres and more than thirty-thousand volunteer members from 130 countries contributing to the Cochrane Library, keeping thousands of reviews up to date, with the goal of providing high-quality, bias-free medical information. Peter Gøtzsche aside its other projects to get the work done, hoping it would lead to new funding. Without having researched mammography before, Gøtzsche's team knew little about the randomized trials that prompted the establishment of Sweden's screening program. But as they assimilated the data, they were baffled. They had expected the trials to be more convincing, but instead they discovered many uncertainties. That made them hurry to get their report done in time for it to be useful in the vote. They delivered it in just four weeks. The team concluded that the scientific basis for introducing screening was "very uncertain," and they could not exclude "the possibility that screening did more harm than good." One of the things they found puzzling was that when they looked at deaths from all causes, as opposed to deaths from only breast cancer, they found more deaths in the women who were screened. Their report cited poor randomization in three of the Swedish trials, discrepancies in numbers between different papers on the same trials, and some women being counted twice. They found much of the data confusing and unreliable.

Gøtzsche presented his eleven-page report a week before the vote in parliament but soon realized that the effort to rush had been futile. It wasn't what the Board of Health, the body proposing to extend screening, wanted the politicians to hear. In his 2012 book *Mammography Screening: Truth, Lies and Controversy*, Gøtzsche details the board's request for changes in his report. Instead of saying the possibility that *screening did more harm than good* could not be excluded, the report would say the possibility that *screening had no effect* could not be excluded. The revised version concluded that it was necessary to undertake a complete Cochrane-style analysis that would seek answers to fundamental questions through contact with all of the trial leaders. Then the board said the report was provisional and would not be made public. Denmark's political leaders did not get a chance to read it and, unaware of what it contained, voted in favour of the plan to extend screening. The vote meant that all local regions could implement programs. Gøtzsche was livid that the Board of Health "preferred to deep-freeze" the report "like a corpse one wants to get rid of before others begin to notice the smell." But the corpse didn't stay in the deep freeze for long. A newspaper journalist learned about the withholding of Gøtzsche's analysis and wrote two front-page articles revealing that the board was suppressing a report that questioned screening's effectiveness. Parliamentarians demanded to know why they weren't entitled to see the information. The board relented and offered the document to anyone who asked for it but distanced itself from the findings.

Gøtzsche was not about to leave it there. The board did agree to fund a full Cochrane review, and that would give him the opportunity to expand his quick four-week investigation and contact all the trial leaders for additional information and data. In the meantime, however, he decided that the world should know about the initial report and, with his colleague Ole Olsen, submitted a paper to the *Lancet*. Its publication in January 2000 incited a new round in the international mammography debate. Until then, the Canadian study was the one most heavily criticized, a constant target for those who believed screening saves lives. Now Gøtzsche applauded the Canadian study and ripped apart the Swedish research the mammographers extolled.

He reviewed all seven of the world's breast-screening trials and dismissed five of them because he judged their randomization poor. In randomized controlled trials, both groups — the group getting a drug or procedure and the control group — must be similar. One group can't be older than the other or less wealthy, smoke more, or exercise less. Individual characteristics are variables that can change the outcome of a study and so should be distributed evenly in both groups. If you're testing a blood pressure drug, for instance, you don't want the drug group to have more young people than the control group, or more participants who exercise or eat better, because any of those factors by themselves could account for lower blood pressure and disguise the true effect of the drug. In breast-screening trials, age is important because the older you are, the greater your risk of breast cancer. Family history of breast cancer is another variable. In the five trials he dismissed, Gøtzsche found that the groups either weren't evenly matched or he couldn't tell if they were because the variables weren't accounted for. The only factor reported in the Swedish trials was age, and average ages in the groups weren't the same. The differences were small, amounting to months rather than years, but even small differences can matter when thousands of people are involved. Another puzzling problem was that in four of the five Swedish trials, the number of women randomized changed in different reports from those trials, with no explanation. It was as if women just disappeared. Gøtzsche was saying clearly the research that had led to screening programs was flawed.

The title of Gøtzsche and Olsen's paper in the *Lancet* paper asked, "Is Screening for Breast Cancer with Mammography Justifiable?" Their answer was no, it is not. Assessing the twelve-year data in the Swedish trials, they found that, at best, screening biennially for twelve years saved only one woman out of a thousand from dying of breast cancer. But the number of women who died from all causes actually increased among the screened women, and that was not accounting for randomization issues that might have affected the results.

The one Swedish trial Gøtzsche rated well for randomization was the Malmö study, published in 1988. The numbers in this study illustrate an important point about the benefits of screening. Researchers randomized forty thousand women over age forty-five living in the city of Malmö to split them evenly into either a group invited to screening or a control group. After ten years, sixty-three of the women in the screened group and sixty-six in the control group had died of breast cancer. Notice first that the number of deaths is small and second that the difference is only three. Other studies indicated that screening had a greater effect in older women, so the researchers looked at the twenty-five thousand women in the study who were over fifty-five. Thirty-five in the screened group and forty-four in the unscreened control group died, a difference of nine.

There are two ways to look at that difference. Statisticians commonly report it as a relative number and would identify a 20 percent reduction in the risk of mortality, referring to the reduction of nine deaths from forty-four. Twenty percent seems like a lot. But the difference can also be expressed as an absolute number that tells us the actual risk.

Among the twenty-five thousand women over fifty-five, half were in the unscreened control group. In absolute numbers, forty-four out of 12,500 died, or 0.35 percent. That translates to a 0.35 percent absolute risk of dying of breast cancer. Compare that to the absolute risk of dying of breast cancer in the screened group: thirty-five out of 12,500 or 0.28 percent. Reducing the number of deaths by nine out of 12,500 reduces the absolute risk by only 0.07 percent.

Using the relative number, 20 percent, makes a good headline or sound bite, but it exaggerates the benefit. To know the whole story, you need to know exactly what the risk is. Suppose you went to buy a winter coat because there was a 20-percent-off sale. Would you make a choice without knowing the original price? Just because there's 20 percent off doesn't mean you can afford the full-length mink coat. To understand the benefit of screening, you need to ask the same question: 20 percent of what?

The Malmö study was not big enough to permit any firm conclusions, and the researchers could say only that mammography screening "may" lead to reduced mortality from breast cancer. That's because their findings were not statistically significant, meaning that the difference of nine deaths could be due to random chance and not to screening. They would need to study the women longer or have many more women involved. But the numbers illustrate some important context in any discussion about a preventive measure. In Malmö, the risk of death in the ten-year period in which the women were followed was tiny. Beyond those ten years? We know the lifetime risk of dying of breast cancer is about 3 percent, which is much smaller than most people think. Ninety-seven out of a hundred women will die of something else. For some, even though the risk is small, reducing it through screening is simply not debatable. Gøtzsche thinks it is.

The Canadian study led by Anthony Miller and Cornelia Baines came out the most favourably in Gøtzsche and Olsen's review. What they reported then Gøtzsche repeats in *Mammography Screening: Truth, Lies and Controversy*. He finds it ironic that the Canadian trial was the one most heavily criticized as it was by far the best documented. He also points out that although the quality of the Canadian mammography was criticized, the tumours detected were, on average, smaller than those in the Swedish Two-County trial. "How were the mammograms inferior?" he asks. He adds that the Canadian trial was also the only one where the participants gave informed consent. He applauds the study's quality control and accuses screening advocates of propagating malicious truths and punishing Miller and Baines for publishing their quality-control data when none of the others have done so. Gøtzsche says that although it is true that the protocol for randomization made it possible to subvert it, he is satisfied that the Bailar and MacMahon investigation found no evidence that such subversion occurred.

When Baines first read Gøtzsche's paper in the *Lancet*, she thought it was "manna from heaven," the first proper summary of breast-screening trial evidence apart from the 1997 NIH consensus conference. Elsewhere, it was not so well received. Six pages of letters to the editor, taking up more space than the original article, debated his conclusions. Radiologist Lázsló Tabár angrily condemned the paper for an "inaccurate summary of evidence," suggesting that it was "not worthy of a moment's consideration."

More controversy followed. Gøtzsche proceeded to conduct his more thorough review, in accordance with the established Cochrane protocol. Inclusion in the Cochrane Library required the approval of the editors in Cochrane's breast cancer group, based in Australia. After delving further into the data, Gøtzsche had a clear picture of the harms screening caused and wanted to include both harms and benefits in his analysis, but the Cochrane editors wouldn't accept his submission as written. The same group had gone out of its way to disown Gøtzsche and Olsen's 2000 *Lancet* article, and now, after more than a hundred emails regarding the content of his review, Gøtzsche felt that the Cochrane editors were stonewalling. He went back to the *Lancet*. Editor-in-chief Richard Horton made a dramatic decision. He not only agreed to publish another paper in October 2001, but he also put Gøtzsche's entire unapproved review on the *Lancet*'s website and then wrote a blistering editorial about how the venerated Cochrane

Collaboration had this time made a serious mistake. He suggested that the breast cancer group's interference impinged on academic freedom and argued that women should expect doctors to secure the best evidence. "At present," Horton wrote, "there is no reliable evidence from large randomized trials to support screening mammography programs." Gøtzsche and Olsen's paper argued that screening does harm by leading to more aggressive treatment, including 20 percent more mastectomies and, overall, a 30 percent increase in the rate of surgery, because screening finds slow-growing tumours that would never cause a problem in a woman's lifetime. In a February 2002 letter to the *Lancet*, the editors of the Cochrane breast cancer group defended themselves against Horton's implication that they were suppressing information, insisting that some of Gøtzsche's conclusions "remained unsupported by data."

This was as dramatic as it gets in the medical world, involving two giants of medical literature, the *Lancet* and Cochrane. It was a good story for the media. But in October 2001, America was still reeling from 9/11, the horrific al Qaeda terrorist attack that killed over three thousand people when two hijacked planes flew into the World Trade Center in New York, a third crashed into the Pentagon, and a fourth crashed to the ground in Pennsylvania. A European skirmish over mammography screening wasn't making the news. Not yet. Finally, Gina Kolata of the *New York Times* interviewed Gøtzsche and wrote a story outlining his criticisms. On December 10, 2001, the paper printed a bold editorial. Gøtzsche had "raised provocative questions that need to be carefully examined by a panel of experts who are independent of the well-entrenched screening industry," it said. "Many experts believe that a thorough analysis would once again endorse the value of mammography," the editorial concluded. "But it would be nice to be sure."

The experts were soon on it. The NCI provides an online cancer database for physicians called PDQ, or Physician Data Query. The PDQ has a screening and prevention editorial board, a panel of independent experts who review research and write summaries for the database. The PDQ provides assessments of evidence. Its role is advisory. It does not set NCI policy, nor does it make recommendations. In January 2002, the PDQ's editorial board, chaired by the statistician Donald Berry, announced that it would rewrite its statement on screening. It had been telling doctors that the evidence suggested that mammograms, starting at age forty, saved lives. Now it was agreeing that the evidence was insufficient. The board wasn't buying Gøtzsche's arguments completely — it had concerns about how he judged the quality of the screening trials — but it recognized that Gøtzsche had raised important questions that needed more discussion.

In spite of the PDQ evaluation, the NCI said it would continue to recommend that women begin mammography screening at age forty. It was no surprise that the American Cancer Society suggested that the Gøtzsche review was not at all persuasive and took the same position as the NCI. That prompted another editorial from the *New York Times* telling both organizations to reconsider because it was imperative that they "re-examine the evidence closely and not simply go into a defensive crouch." One month later, news from the US Preventive Services Task Force added to the barrage of headlines and editorials. The task force had previously endorsed mammography screening starting at age fifty. Tommy Thompson, secretary of health and human services, the task force's overseer, announced in a press release that the task force was extending the recommendation to include women in their forties. Thompson, whose wife had breast cancer and believed a mammogram saved her life, said the federal government was making a clear recommendation: "If you are forty or older, get screened for breast cancer with mammography every one to two years." The *New York Times*, clearly on a campaign, argued in yet another editorial that Thompson was wrong to declare the debate over and wrong to put the "primatur of his office behind" the new recommendation. The task force's full analysis was not yet made public. The editorial accused Thompson of "acting precipitately" in announcing the verdict before the evidence was available. In fact, the full task force report would not be published until several months later, in the *Annals of Internal Medicine*.

Fran Visco's National Breast Cancer Coalition, like other advocacy groups, was getting questions from members. In April 2002, it offered an eight-page question-and-answer primer on its website, with a thorough summary of the research and a strong opinion. "There is insufficient evidence to support blanket recommendations for or against screening mammography in any age group of women," it said. "There are public health interventions that could save more lives and use fewer health care resources than mammography screening programs."

Could things get more confusing?

Gøtzsche's unapproved review sparked the same kind of anxious conversation in Europe, where in many countries, screening programs instituted because of the Swedish studies were part of government health care systems. If Gøtzsche was right, those programs rested on a shaky foundation of faulty research. In response to the uncertainty, the International Agency for Research on Cancer, an agency of the World Health Organization, organized a working group of twenty-four experts from eleven countries to, once again, examine the evidence. In March 2002, the group concluded that although the evidence that screening women aged forty to forty-nine saved lives was limited, the estimated reduction in mortality for women between fifty and sixty-nine was 35 percent. This evaluation did not include the Canadian results regarding women aged fifty to fifty-nine because the Canadian study did not have an unscreened control group. Score one for the screening side.

The international debate culminated in the Global Summit on Mammographic Screening, called for three days in June at the European Institute of Oncology in Milan. All the key organizations were involved, including the World Health Organization, the US Centers for Disease Control and Prevention, the International Union Against Cancer, and the American Cancer Society. Leaders of the screening trials, representatives from screening programs, critics, interested clinicians, and scientists were invited to attend. The summary conclusion on the final day was that mammography reduced deaths by about 20 percent, and there were no grounds for stopping ongoing screening programs, although "unorganized, opportunistic" screening in physicians' offices should be discouraged. Despite presentations on issues such as false positives and overdiagnosis, the summary conclusion made no mention of harms.

Cornelia Baines was an invited speaker. She came away from the summit dismayed that those who exaggerated the benefits of mammography screening seemed in control, whereas information less favourable to screening was ignored. Daniel Kopans, for instance, reported numbers from a mathematical simulation study suggesting that metastatic cancers could be reduced by 80 percent if women were screened every six months. László Tabár claimed screening resulted in a reduction in mortality of up to 63 percent. He had reported that finding in a paper co-authored with Robert Smith, a director of the American Cancer Society, in the society's own journal, *Cancer*. They based this figure on a comparison of breast cancer mortality in different time periods, before and after screening was introduced. Their concoction of numbers made no sense to Peter Gøtzsche, who had dismissed the paper on several counts, most importantly that such a comparison did not account for other factors that could be at play in different time periods.

Donald Berry, the statistician who chaired the PDQ editorial board, was pilloried for his presentation in Milan, and the personal animosity he experienced took him aback. While he spoke, László Tabár argued from the audience. Berry had encountered Tabár's wrath before. Tabár had threatened to sue the PDQ over its revised assessment of screening. Berry felt shunned at the conference, like a leper, and so attacked that he decided not to attend one morning. One of the conference chairs announced publicly that he had slept in, and although he did not mention Berry's name, it was clear whom he meant. Attempts to shame him didn't stop there. A few days after the conference, he received, via email, a three-page letter from the Finnish radiologist Peter Dean, an associate of László Tabár. In a disrespectful and mean-spirited tirade, Dean accused Berry of professional ignorance and unscientific conduct and of keeping up a campaign against early diagnosis because he wanted to stay in the limelight. Deriding him for "sleeping in," he copied about a hundred other people on the email, provoking Berry to retort, "I'm impressed by the size of your 'cc' list. I want to thank you for not including my mother." He found it particularly unsettling that many of the people Dean copied were friends and respected colleagues.

The cockiness of Dean's email reflected the profound divide between screening advocates and skeptics. At the Milan summit, the advocates thought they had succeeded in refuting Gøtzsche and Olsen and controlling the damage. An editorial by the director of epidemiology and biostatistics at the European Institute of Oncology, where the summit took place, stated the opinion less explicitly but was equally unwavering. "There was unanimity," wrote Peter Boyle, that with current evidence, and taking into account the criticisms of the randomized trials, "there were no grounds for stopping ongoing screening programs" or any planned for the future. "The book on screening trials should now be closed," he said. It was important to concentrate now on making screening programs better, finding ways to ensure full participation, and developing new techniques for early detection.

But anyone who thought the book was closed was mistaken. At the Nordic Cochrane Centre, the file remained open. The Cochrane Library had published Gøtzsche's first review of mammography screening in 2001, but without the data on harms of screening contained in the unapproved version on the *Lancet*'s website. Cochrane reviews are constantly updated, so Gøtzsche kept gathering new data, pressing for clearer information about both the risks and the benefits of screening. Finally, in 2006, the Cochrane Library published a more complete version of his review, "Screening for Breast Cancer with Mammography." Again, he determined that the two trials with adequate randomization, the Canadian and Malmö trials, did not find benefit from screening in any age group. Miller and Baines had published updated results for women over fifty in 2000 and for women in their forties in 2002. When Gøtzsche added data from the other trials (excluding one he deemed biased), he concluded that after ten years of follow-up, the relative reduction in mortality was 15 to 20 percent. Twenty percent of the very small risk of dying meant an absolute reduction of 0.05 percent. He calculated the absolute risk of overdiagnosis or overtreatment to be 0.5 percent. In plain English, for every two thousand women over forty invited for screening in a ten-year period, one will have her life prolonged. Ten women who would not have been diagnosed if not screened will be diagnosed as breast cancer patients and will be treated unnecessarily as a result of a mammogram.

Gøtzsche wasn't the first to talk about harms from breast screening. But now he quantified them. The question he posed was: even if screening had some benefit, did the harms outweigh it? "Women, clinicians and policy makers," the Cochrane review summed up, "should consider the trade-offs carefully when they decide whether or not to attend or support screening programs."

That's exactly what the US Preventive Services Task Force attempted to do in 2009, causing yet more mammography pandemonium and confusion and turning another page in a still-open book.

The US Preventive Services Task Force was established in 1984, modelled on the Canadian Task Force on the Periodic Health Examination, created in 1976. The purpose was to assemble a panel of independent experts to determine whether medical practices that were becoming, or had become, routine were predicated on good evidence, specifically practices aimed at preventing disease or detecting it early. Cholesterol tests are an example, as well as blood pressure measurements, colonoscopies, PSA tests, and Pap tests. Much of routine preventive medicine was built on assumptions because clinical trials of preventive measures were few. For example, when doctors thought cholesterol in blood was connected to increased risk of heart disease, they assumed that lowering cholesterol would save lives. Decades later, the effect of lowering cholesterol is still debated, except in people who already have chronic illness, such as diabetes. There has never been a randomized controlled trial to prove that colonoscopies save lives. PSA tests were introduced without a randomized trial.

The Canadian and US task forces aimed to provide clinical guidelines to doctors based on the best evidence available. At first, they published big books containing dozens of guidelines; the Canadian version was known as the "red brick." As the process developed, it became one of ongoing review, with guidelines published one at a time. The

US Preventive Services Task Force protocol is to review each guideline every five years. It had last dealt with mammography screening in 2002, so in 2007, it was time to tackle this impossible, irresolvable issue yet again.

The process took many months more than expected. The task force had to look at other screening methods besides mammography, such as breast self-exams and clinical breast exams, and new technology, such as MRI tests. Working groups took different topics and would report back to the larger group, largely in telephone conference calls. While task force members sifted through old data and past task force reviews, an outside research group looked at all the new evidence. All sixteen task force members were volunteers and received no compensation. Ned Calonge, a physician and public health specialist from Colorado, was the chair, and like other chairs of such panels dealing with breast screening, he was not prepared for the passionate politics that would confront him.

As before, the controversy was around screening women under age fifty. The 2002 task force had recommended screening for women in their forties but noted "the precise age at which the benefits from screening mammography justify the potential harms is a subjective judgment and should take into account patient preferences." The task force said clinicians needed to inform patients of both the benefits and the risks. But oddly, the recommendation, even though seemingly equivocal, had a high rating. The way a recommendation is rated tells you something about the strength of the evidence behind it. Recommendations earn an A rating for high certainty of substantial benefit, B for high certainty of moderate benefit or moderate certainty of high benefit, and C if the benefit of a preventive service is small, in which case, a service, such as screening, should be offered selectively. A D rating means that it's not recommended. The 2002 recommendation for screening women in their forties was rated B even though it failed to clearly set out what doctors should tell their patients.

As the new chair and new members of the task force began the process of updating the screening recommendations, they had Gøtzsche's

Cochrane review to consider along with their own analysis of the latest data. Their assessments differed from the Cochrane research in many respects, and Gøtzsche hadn't concerned himself with the differences between women over or under fifty. But what the task force ended up saying was equally controversial. On Monday, November 16, 2009, it recommended against routine screening for women in their forties, encouraging individualized, informed decision making about when to begin screening. It was a C recommendation. The task force said screening reduced mortality by 15 percent for women in their forties and by 17 percent (relative number) for women aged fifty to sixty-nine. However, the balance of harm was greater in the forty-to-forty-nine age group.

Calonge recalls that a press release had been written but was never issued, and he never learned why. Media were left on their own to decipher the task force's report in the *Annals of Internal Medicine* or on the task force website. When Calonge tuned in to the news on his car radio the day the report was released, he heard the task force was recommending against mammograms. Newspapers told the same story the next day. But the task force did not recommend against mammograms for all women under fifty; it said it could not recommend "routine" mammograms and the decision to begin screening should be an individual one depending on the patient's values regarding benefits and harms. It wasn't much different in tone than the 2002 recommendations — and not much clearer. But the subtleties were lost, and reaction was swift. Kathleen Sebelius, secretary of health and human services, immediately issued a strong statement distancing the federal government from the recommendations. "There is no question that the US Preventive Services Task Force recommendations have caused a great deal of confusion and worry among women and their families across this country," she said. "I want to address that confusion head-on." The task force, she pointed out, didn't make policy and didn't determine what services federal health plans covered.

The phones in Calonge's office lit up. Reporters hounded task force members. The one member who was somewhat prepared was the vice-chair and spokesperson for the panel, Diana Petitti. Some media had access to the recommendations ahead of time, under embargo, and Petitti could tell from the reporters' questions they hadn't understood what the task force was saying. She also sensed much more than the usual interest, and very soon their demands overwhelmed her. Petitti, a physician and epidemiologist who loves numbers, was at Arizona State University while volunteering her time on the task force. She had to drop everything for a few weeks and designate someone in her university office to take phone calls. She remembers a Saturday morning when, still in pyjamas, she watched a news van come up her driveway just as the phone rang. Someone was calling her to warn that the reporter, already there, was coming. Missives from an angry public accompanied the onslaught of media queries. One person threatened to get her fired from her job. Another sent a death threat. She received emails from people who accused her of killing their mothers. The university had to put on extra security. The American College of Radiology had mobilized spokespersons ready with talking points in the major media market, and Petitti was surprised at the hostility in the organization's press release attacking the credentials of the people on the task force. She thought the radiologists were hysterical. Calonge was just hanging on until Thanksgiving, a little more than a week away, hoping that after the holidays, people would start thinking about other things. Panel members stopped accepting media calls and invitations to television studios. "We just decided we'd lost the media," Calonge explains. "There was nothing we could say on air, and really, all the TV folks wanted was someone for a woman to be yelling at. So we just refused everything."

Complicating matters was the business of the C rating for the controversial recommendation. The report was released just days before a Senate vote on the Affordable Care Act, better known as Obamacare. Calonge and the task force were unaware that the legislation was going to reference their recommendations. The Affordable Care Act said full payment for preventive services, such as mammography screening, without a patient having to co-pay would, at a minimum, apply to those with B or higher recommendations. The act said nothing about recommendations below B. It was about setting a floor, not a ceiling, and insurers could continue to pay for breast screening of younger women or ask for partial payment from the patient. The immediate reaction to the task force recommendation, however, was that women under fifty were going to be forced to pay for their mammograms, and if they couldn't afford them, it would mean that they didn't have an equal chance at life. The task force was a death panel, politicians cried, catastrophic for women's health.

Calonge and Petitti were immediately called to testify in Congress, where it became clear that they were pawns in a political fight. For Petitti, that was the worst thing of all. She spent a sleepless Thanksgiving weekend worrying about how she would handle what she anticipated would be a hostile environment. For four gruelling hours, she and Calonge tried to defend the science behind the task force recommendations. She was visibly nervous, stumbling over her prepared statement. But she soon realized that this congressional committee debate had little to do with science, nothing to do with the information she could offer, and everything to do with political posturing. The Democrats said the idea that mammograms wouldn't be paid for was preposterous. The Republicans were using the breast-screening recommendation as a reason not to support the Democrats' health care reform. For the two doctors, it was a hard political lesson. Petitti admitted that she had been naively oblivious to the details of the reform package. Calonge was vaguely aware of them, but he did not know the task force recommendations would be at play. Petitti also acknowledged that they had communicated poorly and should have had a formal communications plan to reach both consumers and physicians.

Politics aside, the task force had made a bold declaration, not so much in its precise recommendations but by demonstrating the weakness of the evidence for screening women, even in their fifties. The task force looked at the same randomized trials Gøtzsche and his team had reviewed for Cochrane. Although they interpreted the data differently, they both pointed out that every study, including the Canadian one, had limitations. The evidence for and against screening was still unclear, and in that sense, the task force gave significant weight to Gøtzsche's work as well as Miller and Baines's. It concluded that screening reduces deaths by 15 percent — hardly a triumphant number. Today, Calonge says even if you accept an estimate of 25 percent, it's still poor, especially if you think about how we approach a lot of other medicine. "It's always bothered me that we're not looking for some other approach," he says. "All the eggs are in the mammography basket."

The political problem was rooted in a proposed stipulation of the Affordable Care Act that insurance coverage for certain services such as mammography screening be tied to the grades the US Preventive Services Task Force assigned to its recommendations. In the end, Congress legislated an exception for breast screening so that women had a right to free mammograms without any co-payment. This was partly due to lobbying from radiologists, who argued that women under fifty should not face a financial barrier to screening.

Peter Gøtzsche continued to update his Cochrane review, publishing the most recent version in 2013. Today, he's even more doubtful about the benefits of mammography screening, suggesting that a 15 percent reduction in mortality is optimistic and the rate of overdiagnosis is higher than first thought. Such poor results from a drug, he says, would be entirely unacceptable. Mortality from breast cancer has gone down, most likely because of better treatment, not screening; it's down even in countries where no screening exists. His message to women is that they need to be aware of the limitations of early detection and the risks of overdiagnosis, and he continues to say screening should stop.

At the end of an eventful decade, Anthony Miller and Cornelia Baines could feel a measure of vindication from Gøtzsche's work and from the US Preventive Services Task Force's extensive review and its recommendations. The National Breast Cancer Coalition, representing a powerful group of women with breast cancer, was on their side, as was the Washington-based lobby, the National Women's Health Network.

The work of other scientists around the world was providing a better understanding of overdiagnosis. But the religion of early detection was still guiding public health policy, and the debate over screening was far from over. Miller and Baines would find themselves in the mammography maelstrom once more.

Nine   SLINGS AND ARROWS

When Cornelia Baines told her eightieth birthday party guests she suffered "not from the slings and arrows of outrageous fortune, but from the slings and arrows of outraged radiologists," she was fresh from a new round in the mammogram wars. The latest volley of slings and arrows from radiologists had begun in February 2014, when she, Anthony Miller, and others published a twenty-five-year follow-up of the Canadian National Breast Screening Study in the *BMJ*. It was front-page news, and, indeed, radiologists were outraged.

Miller and Baines had last reported on their data in 2000 and 2002, concluding again that mammography screening had no benefit for women in their forties and no benefit greater than a clinical breast examination for women in their fifties. But Miller still had a niggling question: what if mammography proved to have an effect on mortality if the women were studied for a greater length of time? Without longer follow-up, he wasn't content to say there was no benefit. So although he had retired from the University of Toronto and had moved on first to the NCI in the United States and then to the International Agency for Research on Cancer in Lyon and the German Cancer Research Center in Heidelberg, he hung on to the idea of having another look at the Canadian study's data. He eventually secured funding and enlisted the help of Steven Narod, a senior scientist at Women's College Research Institute in Toronto, along with Baines and the other members of the original team.

The screening phase of the study began in 1980. Ninety thousand women between the ages of forty and fifty-nine were recruited in fifteen centres across the country. Among the fifty thousand women under age fifty, half were given mammograms plus clinical breast exams annually for four or five years. The half in the control group were not screened. Among the forty thousand women over fifty, half were allocated to both mammograms and clinical breast exams and half were assigned only to clinical exams. For their 2014 analysis, Miller and colleagues combined the two parts of the study so that the mammography group included all the women screened by both mammography and clinical exams and the control group, the non-mammography group, included all the women who either had no exam or had only clinical exams. Miller would later be criticized for rolling the two age groups into one, but in the *BMJ* paper, the authors explained that they did so because the results either way were similar.

They looked at breast cancer incidence and mortality recorded among all women in the study to the end of 2005. First, they counted only the breast cancers detected during the screening phase and found 666 invasive breast cancers in the mammography group and 524 among the controls. After twenty-five years, 180 of those women in the screened group and 171 in the control group had died. Then they counted all the breast cancers detected in the two groups, both during the screening phase and through the entire follow-up period. By the end of 2005, cancers in the mammography group totalled 3,250, and 500 women had died. Cancers in the control group totalled 3,133, and 505 women had died. The conclusion was clear: for the women in the Canadian study, mammography screening made no impact on breast cancer mortality.

With the updated data, Miller and the team also calculated the rate of overdiagnosis, the number of cancers detected by mammography that would not have caused any symptoms or health problems if never noticed. At the beginning of a randomized trial, there will be more cancers in the screened group because mammography detects the cancers earlier. But after a long enough period of time, the number of cancers detected later in the control group should catch up. There should be the same number of cancers in both the screened group and the unscreened group. A greater number of cancers in the screened group suggests that some were overdiagnosed. The math gets a little complicated here. During the screening phase, there was an excess of 142 invasive breast cancer cases in the screened group — the difference between 666 and 524. After fifteen years, there was still a difference of 106, and that number remained constant through ten more years. To calculate how many cancers were overdiagnosed, it's necessary to understand that among the 666 cancers in the mammography group, 484 were detected at screening. The other cancers were interval cancers, detected during the period between the annual screens. Of the 484 screen-detected cancers, the 106 excess cancers represent 22 percent — the rate of over-diagnosis among the women in the mammography screening group. One in five invasive cancers detected by screening likely did not need the treatment that inevitably followed. That meant, the authors explained, one overdiagnosed breast cancer for every 424 women who received mammography screening during the trial. (Baines, To, and Miller re-evaluated the data in 2016 to include non-invasive cancers known as ductal carcinoma in situ [DCIS] and concluded that the rate of overdiagnosis, including DCIS, was 40 percent in women aged forty to forty-nine and 30 percent in women aged fifty to fifty-nine.)

Predictably, the 2014 update kindled a huge new flare-up in the mammography debate. "Vast Study Casts Doubts on Value of Mammo-grams," headlined Gina Kolata's front-page *New York Times* story. "One of the largest and most meticulous studies of mammography ever done," Kolata began, "has added powerful new doubts about the value of the screening test for women of any age." Similar stories appeared in media around the world, and screening proponents rushed to do what they had always done: attempt to discredit the study. "Shoddy Canadian Research Is Putting Women's Lives at Risk," was the headline for a *Vancouver Sun* opinion piece published two days after the *BMJ* release. "Every credible scientific study supports screening," the author, Paula Gordon, a Vancouver radiologist, wrote. "All, that is, except one, a poorly designed, poorly executed Canadian study that was completed decades ago using outdated mammography machines and corrupted methodology."

The *BMJ* provides a platform for debate on its online site, where readers can send "Rapid Responses," electronic letters to the editor that are vetted and published at the journal's discretion, usually within a day. The Canadian National Breast Screening Study's twenty-five-year follow-up generated sixty-seven such responses. The exchange between supporters of screening and those who question it was vigorous and instructive, but old enemies also made broadside attacks. Harvard radiologist Daniel Kopans repeated the decades-old accusation that improper randomization placed more women with advanced cancers in the screened group. He neglected to mention the independent review of the randomization that cleared the Canadians of any impropriety. He also reiterated the accusation of poor-quality mammography, asserting that the study should have been "disqualified" long ago as a "legitimate" trial. Radiologist László Tabár argued in his lengthy response that "the Canadian trials are uniquely poorly designed and carried out" and were "a failure from the beginning." (Curiously, although the authors of these response letters are required to declare competing interests, Tabár declared that he had none, even though he was the chief executive officer of a private company in Arizona called Mammography Education, Inc., which provides worldwide mammography training. He also advised medical imaging companies.)

Not all radiologists dismissed the Canadian study. John Keen, who practises in Chicago, asked how the quality of the study's mammography could be questioned when it found non-palpable tumours with an average size of 1.4 centimetres, whereas an American survey of screening mammography a few decades later found that the average size typically detected was larger, at 1.8 centimetres. Miriam Pryke, a PhD student at King's College London, commented on the conflicting interpretations. "Data that cannot clinch the matter is no basis for a screening program," she wrote. She declared a competing interest: "diagnosed through screening." Several other experts also came to the defence of Miller and Baines, and their arguments suggest that the

Canadians are not the outliers Kopans and Tabár depict them to be. Miller and Baines took part in the online debate with several letters of their own to answer questions and quarrel with any misinterpretation or errors they felt their critics had made. But they also had to deal with the "slings and arrows" flung at them privately.

On March 4, 2014, three weeks after the report in the *BMJ*, Baines sat down at her computer, opened her email, and recoiled. Waiting in her inbox was a series of three emails, all from "mammomike," all sent within less than half an hour. "Good morning Cornelia," read the first. "We are thoroughly shocked by your recent article published in the *BMJ*." It went on to say that due to the "faulty design and manipulative execution," the Canadian trial should be given no credence. In her defence of the study in the *BMJ* debate, Baines had compared the Canadian trial with László Tabár's study in Sweden. Now mammomike's email told her, "Your study is such an embarrassment to the scientific world that your attempt to compare it with the Swedish Two-County Trial borders on obscenity." Anthony Miller received the same email.

Mammomike is Michael Linver, a radiologist who at the time practised in Albuquerque, New Mexico. The email included several attachments, all negative comments about the Canadian study, including one sent to the *New York Times* in response to Gina Kolata's story, in which Linver described the study as "garbage in, garbage out." He congratulated the newspaper for its "latest contribution to the premature deaths and unnecessary suffering of untold numbers of young women who will contract breast cancer in the next few years." Linver charged that the coverage of the Canadian research was biased and concluded, "The consequent blood on your hands will likely never wash out."

Linver had sent the second email eleven minutes after the first. "Congratulations on all the harm you have done women worldwide. May you never forget it." He included a link to "a lovely video" he thought Baines would enjoy. It was part of an interview Tabár had done for an amateurish-looking social media program called *Breast Cancer Answers*. Apparently not satisfied, Linver sent a third email. "Good morning yet again," he wrote. This time he attached a link to another segment from the same video, in which Tabár denounced the Canadian research.

Four days later, mammomike popped up again with an email addressed to both Baines and Miller. "May the faces of the thousands of women who have died, and will continue to die, prematurely because of you, continue to haunt you in your dreams, and in your nightmares," he wrote.

Linver included László Tabár's name along with his own in the sign-off on each email. The first email mammomike sent, along with his email to the *New York Times*, is posted on Tabár's company's website, in a section that strongly criticizes the Canadian study. Linver says now he doesn't remember whether Tabár helped to write the emails but says they had a lot of discussion. Their professional relationship goes back a long time, Linver recalls, to when he enrolled in the first mammography course Tabár gave in the United States in 1985. "I can tell you that after the first five minutes it was like I had an epiphany, that this was what I wanted to do for the rest of my life. He is so dynamic. He is so charismatic. He's so brilliant." Linver applied Tabár's teachings to this own work in Albuquerque and was so impressed by the increased numbers of small cancers he found that he convinced everyone else in his practice group to also take the course. He speaks with grateful admiration of the huge influence his friend Tabár has had on his life as his mentor and teacher. Linver has also become a mammography trainer and, although retired from practice, still travels the world, spending about twenty weeks a year on the road. He's counted thirteen hundred talks so far, and over the years, he's participated in Tabár's courses on numerous occasions.

Linver is a devout advocate of early detection. He's dedicated his life to mammography, at the expense of music and photography and other things he loves, he says, because it's the way he hopes to make a difference in the world. His passion is his excuse for the angry emails. "It was very emotional for us because basically we'd given our lives to this and so what happened was very upsetting," he says. In one way, he's sorry he wrote them, but he doesn't regret what he said because he thinks it's true. It makes no sense to him that anyone would doubt that screening saves lives. He's said controversial things in his career, he admits in a voice tinged with remorse, and maybe he went a little overboard. "I think we all do that when we're angry," he says. "I don't believe in being silent when I see women dying who I know shouldn't be."

Hurtful mail is hard to receive, even when you've heard the sentiments before, as Baines and Miller had many times. But they've developed thick hides from the decades of defending their work at countless conferences and debates. The slings and arrows from Linver and Tabár are just something they've had to bear. Baines finds it saddening that smart people would react with such hostility and incivility instead of engaging in meaningful discourse. She and Miller feel strongly that they have a duty, as academics, to share their research and talk about it, and they have never had qualms about subjecting their work to close scrutiny. So it should be no surprise that, in 2015, they agreed to walk right into their antagonists' lair, thanks to a professor of radiology in Chicago.

A radiologist since 1963, Leonard Berlin is a senior statesman in the field, a well-respected recipient of honours from the American College of Radiology, among others, for his contributions to the profession. He's a thin, wiry man with a winning smile and a friendly handshake; it's easy to see why he's popular with colleagues. Long ago, he grew interested in malpractice issues, and he is best known for his work in helping radiologists avoid them. Back in the 1970s and 1980s, he recalls, delay in diagnosing breast cancer was one of the most frequent causes of medical malpractice. But as Berlin looked into the issue, he started to think radiologists were overselling mammography and it simply wasn't as good as radiologists wanted patients to believe. He's not against mammography screening, but he believes women have not been getting the whole truth about the negatives and has a distaste for some of the zealous views held by colleagues who dismiss the problem of overdiagnosis. He's published several papers arguing that radiologists have a vested financial interest in breast screening and therefore have been blind to its limitations and perpetrated what he calls the "mammography muddle." He calls for a more open-minded public discussion.

One of his articles got Baines's attention, and she got in touch. An email conversation developed. Berlin likes to attend the Stratford and Shaw festivals in Ontario every year, and after he and his wife included a visit with Baines on one of those trips, they became good friends. After the *BMJ* published the twenty-five-year update of the Canadian study, he got an idea. The American Roentgen Ray Society, an organization of radiologists that draws three to five thousand members to its annual meeting every year, would have its 2015 meeting in Toronto, where Baines and Miller live. There was plenty of controversy. Why not have a debate?

The "Third Annual Great Debate: Mammography Screening Controversies," as it was billed, was the opening event of the week-long conference, beginning at eight a.m. on Sunday, April 19. Miller and Baines were on one side. On the other, Daniel Kopans was teamed with radiologist Paula Gordon, whose scathing opinion piece about the Canadian study appeared in the *Vancouver Sun*. Gordon is a professor of radiology at the University of British Columbia and medical director of the breast program at BC Women's Hospital; she also works with the BC screening mammography program. Just over sixty, she's a relative newcomer to the politics of mammography compared to the other three in the debate. Her introduction was the raucous 1997 NIH consensus conference, which she attended out of interest. She is dark-haired, youthful, tailored, and pert, a striking contrast to the slightly rumpled Kopans.

During the months preceding the Great Debate, Cornelia Baines spent a lot of time preparing her presentation, with assistance from her son on the graphics and visuals. She was well aware that the crowd she'd be speaking to already had strong opinions that she couldn't expect to budge. It wasn't an event she looked forward to. Still, it was important to do a good job. That crisp April morning, she was the first of the celebrated speakers to arrive, in the company of her husband, Andrew; her children, Nicole and Nigel; and her friend, Leonard Berlin. Room

701A at the Metro Toronto Convention Centre is a typically lifeless meeting hall on a subterranean floor, with capacity for five hundred. The room was empty when the Baines entourage walked in. In the awkward, fidgety moments before the audience, or even the other speakers, arrived, Andrew Baines looked at what his wife was wearing: a loose-fitting, stylish jacket in striking red, black sweater and pants, and, slung over her shoulder, a small lime-green purse. "Did you mean to choose that one?" he asked. "Yes," she replied. "Sometimes I like to be flamboyant on purpose. So that I am less intimidated."

Anthony Miller walked into the room, unaccompanied, not long after. Dressed smartly in a dark suit, he showed no sign that he was even a little intimidated. It wasn't the most fun thing to be doing so early on a Sunday, but he had been on the same stage as Daniel Kopans many times before. Kopans and Gordon also arrived well ahead of time, as they had been asked to, and the two camps milled about as they waited for the audience to arrive.

The two-hour event had been carefully planned. Each speaker was allotted a strict fifteen minutes to present and then some time for rebuttals. Questions from the floor would follow. Presentation slides had to conform to technical requirements because the debate was live-streamed to Roentgen Ray Society members who couldn't attend in person. Miller spoke first, outlining the data from the Canadian breast screening trial. Baines followed with answers to specific criticisms that had been made about the study over the years. Gordon was next, with a presentation focused on the quality of the study's mammograms. She showed just one mammogram from the Canadian study, one of obviously poor quality, and compared it to a visibly better mammogram from Sweden done at around the same time. She argued that inferior x-rays would explain why the study found no reduction in mortality among the screened women. It was all very polite and impersonal until Kopans got up and opened his fifteen minutes with the declaration that he had not wanted to participate. "Even though Cornelia and Tony think I'm evil," he said, "I'm actually very fond of them." He then made his familiar argument that randomization issues compromised the

Canadian study, and he challenged Miller's estimate of overdiagnosis, suggesting that, according to his own calculation, the rate of overdiagnosis was only 4 percent, not 22 percent.

In his rebuttal, Miller remarked that he had presented the correct analysis based on the data. "I leave it to you to judge who is telling the truth," he told the radiologists in the audience, "those who have access to the data, or those who look from the outside and make these assertions." He also took exception to the slide Gordon had presented. Miller suspected that the one image had come from the very early days of the study in 1980 and had been supplied by Martin Yaffe, who, as the reference physicist, would have been monitoring the films with the express purpose of ferreting out such substandard mammograms. Miller thought it was deceptive to select just this one and not any subsequent films. Miller had shown in his presentation, and now reminded the room, that the Canadian mammograms were, in fact, more sensitive than the Swedish ones, capturing smaller tumours. Although Tabár is widely lauded for his skill at performing mammography and teaching it, Miller noted that there are no data regarding the quality of the mammograms in his study, except for the size of tumours he's reported. Gordon later acknowledged that Yaffe had long ago provided that one mammogram from the Canadian study. She'd been using it in talks for twenty-five years.

In her presentation, Gordon also referenced a 2014 Canadian paper reporting that mammography screening reduces breast cancer mortality by 40 percent. The study by Andrew Coldman, a statistician and emeritus scientist at the BC Cancer Agency, is one screening enthusiasts invariably cite when marshalling their arguments. Coldman and his fellow authors looked at data covering the period from 1990 to 2009 from seven breast screening programs in Canada as well as data from provincial cancer registries. They tabulated breast cancer mortality rates among women who had participated in screening programs at least once. They then estimated the "expected" mortality rate based on the incidence of cancer and survival rates among women who had not participated. They concluded that the mortality rate among screened women was 40 percent lower than expected, and it didn't matter how old the women were when they first went for screening. It may look like a slam dunk for screening, but there are some important issues.

The first thing to understand is that this study was not a randomized controlled trial, in which women were equally distributed into groups with well-matched characteristics. Rather, it was an observational study based only on available statistical data. Comparing screening participants to non-participants is problematic because it can be biased. It's known that people who attend screening programs tend to be wealthier, better educated, and generally healthier than people who don't. This is known as the "healthy screenee" effect. Comparing a screened group to a non-screened group is a little like comparing apples to oranges. A healthy screening bias couldn't alone account for an effect as dramatic as a 40 percent mortality reduction, however. There's another problem. If you were to look carefully at who attends screening programs, you would find it's not people with cancer. People already diagnosed see specialists; they don't have a reason to attend a screening clinic. It's not known how many in the Coldman study already had cancer by 1990 and would have been counted among the non-screened. Another question is, among the women screened, how was their breast cancer detected? The study does not tell us how many cancers were found through screening and how many were found by the women themselves. Also, a database that includes women who've participated in a screening program as little as once, over such a long period of time, casts a wide net that could include those whose breast cancer wasn't discovered until many years after they were screened. Finally, when you find indolent cancers that would not go noticed except for screening, you increase the incidence of cancer, as Cornelia Baines explains, and that makes it look as if you're decreasing the death rate.

Consider, too, that a 40 percent lower mortality rate than expected is one of those vague relative numbers that exaggerate. Forty percent of what? Of what risk? What we do know is that the absolute lifetime risk of dying of breast cancer is low, about 3 percent. Ninety-seven percent of women will die of something else. But a 40 percent reduction in mortality is a catchy statistic, and breast-screening proponents love to flaunt it.

The Great Debate was civil, thanks in part to an effective moderator who cut things off at the right moment to move things along and avoid any rehashing of arguments already made. Terry Minuk, a radiologist from Hamilton, Ontario, stood up to say his hospital assigned him to the Canadian study without any training. In an interview later, Minuk explained that at the time, radiologists in Canada received no special mammography training in medical school. With the help of a few days of immersion with the study's reference radiologist in Toronto, he learned on the job. Today, he is the lead radiologist in the Hamilton region's breast screening program, and mammography is a major part of his work. He credits the breast screening study with dramatically improving the quality of mammography in Canada but says the mammography was poor at the beginning of the study. Roberta Jong, a Toronto radiologist who was also involved in the study and has been a harsh critic, went to the microphone to insist that the randomization in the study could have been subverted, which she believed happened. To critics, it never seems to matter that the Canadian study was audited and exonerated on that score. But the comments were generally respectful, everyone was appropriately applauded for their contributions, and Miller and Baines went home feeling that although they might not have gained any apostles, their own skins were intact, barely grazed by the expected volley of slings and arrows.

The very next day, April 20, 2015, renewed vindication came their way.

The US Preventive Services Task Force, mandated to update its recommendations every five years, had opened a new discussion on screening mammography. On April 20, a year behind schedule, it put forward a draft revision. The public would have a chance to respond before the task force finalized any new recommendations. Kopans knew what was coming and had blurted out what he called a "spoiler alert" at the Great Debate, even though the information was under embargo. "They're going to say, 'Don't screen women in their forties,'" he revealed. "Their decision is based on the Canadian study."

Kopans knew about the draft because someone in the media, allowed to have advance notice and seek expert opinion for a story, contacted him. Sharing the details, as Kopans did at the meeting, was inappropriate, and a member of the audience mildly chastised him for breaking the embargo and cautioned everyone in the room not to put it out on social media. Regardless, both of Kopans's statements were rhetorical oversimplifications and not exactly accurate. The task force would never make recommendations solely on the basis of one study. It would certainly have looked at the new data from Canada published the year before, but it needed to review any available new data, and its reviews are extensive and thorough. Kopans believes the Canadian study should be left out of the process entirely. His message has always been that it shouldn't be considered in any development of public policy.

As for the part about not screening women in their forties, the task force draft did not recommend against screening, contrary to Kopans's claim. In much more nuanced wording, it said, "The decision to start screening mammography in women prior to age fifty years should be an individual one. Women who place a higher value on the potential benefit than the potential harms may choose to begin biennial screening between the ages of forty and forty-nine years." The task force explained that screening women under fifty may reduce the risk of dying of breast cancer, but the harms resulting from false positives and overdiagnosis are greater in this age group than in older women. It rated the recommendation as a C, meaning moderate certainty that the net benefit of screening was small or, in simpler English, the evidence for mass population screening of asymptomatic women is weak, so the task force could not recommend it. But it also did not recommend against it.

In its draft, the task force recommended biennial screening for women ages fifty to seventy-four, a B-rated recommendation indicating moderate certainty of moderate net benefit of screening. In this age group, the most important harm is overdiagnosis; other harms include false positives and false negatives and a small risk of breast cancer resulting from repeated radiation exposure over many years of screening. After analyzing all of the screening trials, it concluded that

The media's subdued response might have had something to do with a much more dramatic event a few months earlier, in October. The American Cancer Society, which had long held the view that women should be screened annually starting at age forty and had vehemently objected to the 2009 task force guidelines, suddenly made a right-hand turn. It announced new recommendations that women should begin screening later and do it less often. Women with an average risk of breast cancer should begin screening at age forty-five and have annual exams until age fifty-five, at which time they should transition to exams every other year. In explaining the reasoning behind the changes, the American Cancer Society said that, in summary, mammography in women aged forty to sixty-nine was associated with a reduction in breast cancer death. But taking harms into consideration, the conclusion was that "a lesser, but not insignificant, burden of disease for women aged 40 to 44 years and the higher cumulative risk of adverse outcomes no longer warranted a direct recommendation to begin screening at age 40 years." It was a huge story that led network evening newscasts and featured prominently in major daily newspapers.

The changes, although seemingly small and subtle, signalled a tectonic shift in thinking from one of the most powerful advocates of screening in the world. The recognition that screening brought harm as well as benefit was significant. The American Cancer Society was saying that population screening based on a one-size-fits-all paradigm might not be the best approach. For decades, one of the staunchest mammography proponents was Robert Smith, the society's director of cancer screening. "I'll be very happy if our guidelines diminish the polarization around this issue," he told AuntMinnie.com. "The hope is that people will really consider these guidelines rather than just defend their entrenched positions." The Berlin Wall of screening was beginning to crumble.

The reaction from proponents such as Daniel Kopans and the American College of Radiology was swift, and predictable. Their view was that women should begin annual breast screening at forty, regardless of what the American Cancer Society had decided. And their spin was that the American Cancer Society was confirming that mammography saved lives, even though recommending a later start.

The society's abrupt change in tone might not have been anticipated at the Great Debate in Toronto just six months earlier. Radiologists' main concern then was that the Canadian screening study might influence the US Preventive Services Task Force. Facing a group that needed to find fault with the Canadian study, Miller and Baines could only do their best, knowing they were unlikely to change anyone's mind. But Baines had something she wanted them all to know. She spoke softly but clearly, standing tall and confident. She came to the end of her presentation and summed up. "Dr. Kopans worries about denying access to screening and claims overdiagnosis is a myth," she said. "I worry about screening doing more harm than good. To be overdiagnosed is to be overtreated, breast cancer treatment is not good for your health, [and] screen detection increases the risk of total mastectomy."

And then, without any pause, she said, "I have breast cancer."

It wasn't said to shock or alarm. Some in the room would already have known about her cancer from reading her description of it in a 2005 *BMJ* opinion piece. It was more a "matter-of-fact way" of pre-empting anyone from saying, "But you don't know what it's like." At the end of the debate, the first person from the audience to ask a question wanted to know how Baines's cancer was diagnosed. She told her story.

Baines had put herself in the National Breast Screening Study and was grateful that she wasn't allocated to the screening group. She was still in her forties. But in her fifties, she felt a "kind of scientific" obligation, on the basis of evidence at the time, to get a mammogram. She did so after the Ontario breast screening program opened in 1991, well after the screening phase in the study ended. When she was sixty, a screening mammogram indicated a lesion in her right breast. Specialists ordered diagnostic mammograms and arranged follow-up in six months. The density of the tumour did not change in that time, and both surgeon and radiologist concluded that she'd had a false positive result.

One morning nine years later, just out of the shower, she noticed something in the mirror. There was a flattening in the right breast, at six o'clock. A diagnostic workup revealed cancer, exactly where something had shown up suspiciously on the earlier mammogram. A false positive had turned into a false negative. Baines had a lumpectomy and was sent for radiation, but she stopped the therapy before it was over when her chronic kidney problem flared. No lymph node involvement and a tumour that was ER-positive and had clean margins indicated a good prognosis. Although one regular follow-up exam indicated something suspicious, it turned out not to be, and she's been clear of breast cancer since.

Was she frightened? No, she says. She didn't like it, but she was not terrified by the diagnosis. The science told her most people don't die of breast cancer, and she received the appropriate therapy. She also knew from life experience that no one could predict what would happen to her. She had been there before. When she was a young woman, she didn't expect to survive the lymphoma that caused her to put aside her medical training for a few years. She's also had thyroid cancer, probably due to the radiation she received for the lymphoma. Add *stoic* to the list of adjectives that describe Cornelia Baines. She'll answer questions about her health but won't linger on the details. She prefers to rejoice in the fulfillments of life: her family and friends, her music, her farm, and the privilege of continuing to do stimulating and interesting work, slings and arrows notwithstanding.

Ten   IS IT EVEN CANCER?

Therese Taylor was fifty-two when she had her first clinical breast exam, in the office of a new family doctor. He recommended that she go for a mammogram. After she shrugged the suggestion off, protesting that she wasn't interested, he told her he'd found a lump in her right breast. Suddenly, she was confronting the thing that every woman dreads. So she complied. She went for the mammogram a few days later, in the first week of October 2011. No lump in the right breast was visible on the x-ray. Little white specks showed up in several places in the image of the left breast, however, flecks of calcium that flag the presence of malignant cells. These "microcalcifications" meant that she needed to see a surgeon. Ten slow, anxious days after a biopsy, the surgeon had her back in his office and gave her the diagnosis. She had DCIS.

DCIS is diagnosed when malignant cells are confined within the milk ducts of the breast. When a tumour breaks through the walls of the ducts and invades surrounding tissue, it becomes invasive breast cancer. On a mammogram, DCIS can look like a string of calcium specks, sometimes lined up in linear fashion, sometimes following a squiggly path, and sometimes spread more diffusely, in a feather-like pattern. It can occur in different parts of the same breast. The calcium results from cancer cells dying off. Sometimes DCIS is a solid tumour within the milk duct but rarely is large enough to feel, and because it's not palpable, almost all DCIS is diagnosed as a result of a mammogram. The condition was first described a century ago by the surgeon and pathologist Joseph Colt Bloodgood at Johns Hopkins University, but it was only when mammography screening started to become popular in the 1980s that DCIS was routinely detected. Because of mammography, the incidence of DCIS in the United States increased more than sevenfold from the mid-1970s to the end of the 1990s. Today, it's estimated that between 20 and 30 percent of cancers detected in screening mammograms are DCIS. In the United States, over fifty thousand new cases of DCIS are diagnosed every year, most in women between the ages of fifty and sixty.

Yet it's not clear what DCIS really is. Historically, DCIS has been considered a precancerous condition, a precursor of invasive cancer, in the way that some suspicious cells in the cervix discovered in a Pap test are considered precancerous. Therefore, to prevent DCIS from becoming invasive, the standard protocol is to excise it. This practice is becoming increasingly controversial because most DCIS will not progress to invasive cancer, but the difficulty is knowing which ones will and when. So multitudes of women are undergoing lumpectomies and, depending on how widespread the DCIS is in the breast, full mastectomies for a poorly understood and unpredictable precancerous condition that might not cause any harm. Is it even fair to call it precancer? Some experts argue that it isn't and that calling it a carcinoma is mislabelling if not misleading. Thanks to mammography screening, the ability to detect DCIS is contributing to overdiagnosis.

Therese Taylor didn't know any of this when her surgeon told her she needed to have her breast removed. DCIS was "consistent with cancer," he said. She didn't ask him to explain what he meant, thinking it was just a nice way of saying "You've got cancer." She went home dazed by the news. Taylor returned for a second consultation a few days later, this time with her husband, and asked what stage her cancer was. "Stage zero," the surgeon said. Taylor didn't think to ask what that meant either. The surgeon said he was pretty sure she wouldn't need radiation or chemotherapy, but she had to have a mastectomy because the DCIS appeared to be in too wide an area to capture with a simple lumpectomy. "It was numbing," Taylor says. "The worst part was telling the kids and wondering how worried about it they were going to be."

Taylor had been living a comfortable life in a spacious suburban house in Mississauga, Ontario. When she was diagnosed, her eldest son was in college, the younger one was in high school, and her daughter was twelve. The family moved to Mississauga in 2002, when the house was relatively new, built less than fifteen years before. They loved the mature trees in the backyard, surprised by their presence in such a young neighbourhood. Taylor learned that her home was in a residential development carved out of an old Carolinian forest, and tree preservation had been a condition of construction. But some of the trees were dying because people had been choking them with lawns. Taylor called in an expert to help her save the ash and shagbark hickory trees highlighting the view from her kitchen and dining area, and she replaced an expanse of grass with a bird-welcoming garden of shrubs and native plants. Soon she was leading a fight at city hall to save a two-hectare woodland nearby.

Soft-spoken, small in stature, and dressed conservatively in brown, Taylor gives the impression of someone entirely unassuming. She's not a person you'd notice in a crowd. Her long brown hair hangs below her shoulders, with a fringe that frames a small face that is warm but with an earnestness that suggests a person who has convictions. The compliance with which she obeyed her surgeon seems at odds with the determined way she set about to save trees, but it all happened fast. Taylor received her diagnosis on October 28. She had the mastectomy two weeks later, on November 14. Three weeks after the operation, she saw the surgeon once more so that he could check on her wound. That was the first time she heard the word *precancer*.

A few years after the mastectomy, Taylor heard something on the radio about overdiagnosis of breast cancer and, later that night, saw a television news story. She needed to know more and launched into research. One of the first things she came across was a 2009 Associated Press story in the *Toronto Star* headlined "Milk Duct Tumours Not Really Cancer." The story was about a comprehensive report from the NIH attempting to sort out the controversy, confusion, and uncertainty around DCIS.

In September 2009, leading breast cancer researchers had gathered at the Natcher Conference Center on the NIH campus to review and discuss the current science around detecting and treating DCIS. At the end of the four-day meeting, they issued what they titled the "State-of-the-Science Conference Statement on Diagnosis and Management of Ductal Carcinoma in Situ." A DCIS patient would not get much comfort from the twenty-page document noting that "the natural history of DCIS is poorly understood" and management and diagnosis of it are highly complex. Many unanswered questions remained, the researchers said. Most vexing was (and still is): how can we know when DCIS will develop into invasive breast cancer? Pathologists had determined that there are different "grades" of DCIS depending on the patterns created by the proliferation of cancer-like cells and how densely packed they are within the duct. The most worrisome is high grade, when the cells become compacted enough to plug the duct, and the cells in the centre become starved of nourishment and die, resulting in what's called comedo necrosis. The evidence was that high-grade DCIS was "strongly associated" with the risk of developing invasive breast cancer. But an association is not cause and effect. Rather, it's an observation that two things are happening at the same time and are possibly connected. Nor was the science strong enough to say only women with high-grade DCIS should be treated.

And what should the treatment be? Breast-conserving surgery (lumpectomy)? Full mastectomy? Lumpectomy combined with radiation? Drugs such as tamoxifen, sometimes used to prevent invasive cancer? The questions the scientists were trying to answer in 2009 still have no definitive answers. The standard of care for DCIS today, as then, calls for surgery. If it's contained in a small area, a simple lumpectomy might suffice, and sometimes that's done along with a procedure to check for any immediate involvement of lymph nodes. But if it is spread out to the point that a lumpectomy would remove so much tissue that it would be cosmetically unacceptable, a complete mastectomy is standard. Mastectomies are done in about a quarter of DCIS cases.

Therese Taylor's DCIS was classified as high grade and was detected in more than one place in her breast. Her surgeon was following the protocol of the time and probably what he understood to be best for his patient. She doesn't understand, however, why there was such a hurry. She feels she was coerced, first by the family physician who persuaded her to go for a mammogram, even though she herself couldn't feel the lump he said he'd found, and again by the surgeon who rushed her to the operating room, leading her to believe invasive disease threatened her life.

Taylor opted not to undergo another surgery for breast reconstruction, so she lives with a scar across her left breast that is a constant reminder of a loss she feels deeply, not with anger but with sadness. For a long time, she wore her hair long enough so that she could brush it down over her disfigurement. "Don't look down," she would tell herself as she stood in the shower. "Don't look down."

Taylor feels that if she had known there was a controversy and understood more about the condition, she might have made a different choice. She certainly would have thought about it longer. For her, the NIH report on DCIS was an eye-opener.

The NIH state-of-the-science panel consisted of fourteen members representing oncology, radiology, surgery, obstetrics and gynecology, epidemiology, biostatistics, pathology, nursing, preventive medicine, and social work. In addition, twenty-two experts were invited to speak to the panel. Karla Kerlikowske was one of the first, there to discuss the prevalence of DCIS. Kerlikowske is a physician in internal medicine and professor of medicine specializing in epidemiology and biostatistics at the University of California, San Francisco. She has published widely on breast imaging, the epidemiology of invasive breast cancer, DCIS, and predicting the risk of invasive breast cancer. This wasn't her first appearance at the Natcher Conference Center; she was one of the speakers at the infamous 1997 NIH consensus development conference on mammography screening for women aged forty to forty-nine. She recalls with giddy excitement in her voice that, on that occasion, she was lucky enough to sit next to the revered Sam Shapiro, the epidemiologist who designed the foundational New York HIP study. "He was such a sweet man," she says. "Just a doll." Her task was to review the results from his trial, and all of the other trials, pertinent to screening women in their forties. There was no evidence, she observed then, that screening women in that age group had any impact on mortality.

Twelve years later, she was back at the NIH, expressing alarm about DCIS. Kerlikowske told the panel screening mammography had led to a DCIS "epidemic." Somewhere between 17 and 34 percent of all breast cancer cases found through mammography were DCIS. Yet despite twenty years of detecting DCIS on mammograms, the incidence of invasive breast cancer had not declined. A decrease in the incidence of invasive breast cancer had been seen only briefly once, after women abruptly stopped taking hormone replacement therapy, or HRT. Evidence had suggested that HRT protected women against both heart disease and osteoporosis, so in 1993, the Women's Health Initiative of the NIH began a trial of almost seventeen thousand women to investigate the long-term health effects of taking a combination of estrogen and progesterone. But in 2002, the NIH abruptly stopped the trial, three years before it was supposed to end, because those randomized to take HRT had a higher incidence of breast cancer than those randomized to placebo. The bombshell caused an immediate, widespread abandonment of HRT. A distinct drop in new breast cancer cases followed. It was the only change observed in two decades. If early detection of DCIS worked, it should have resulted in consistently fewer cases of invasive cancer, and that wasn't happening.

Kerlikowske is articulate and plainspoken, and she addresses a crowd in the way that you imagine she might speak to a patient, clearly and confidently. She has a reassuring smile and punctuates her speech with an occasional little laugh, almost but not quite a giggle. In a lecture for the University of California's mini medical school, shortly before the NIH panel on DCIS, she provided a detailed but accessible breakdown of what scientists knew. The essential facts haven't changed. Only 15 percent of DCIS cases progress to invasive cancer within ten years. Even more encouraging, only 2 percent of women treated for DCIS will die within ten years. Kerlikowske suggests that means one of two things: either the surgery and treatments for DCIS are effective or indolent malignancies that would never cause harm are being treated unnecessarily. In the absence of clinical trials comparing women treated for DCIS to a control group of untreated women, it isn't possible to determine which of the two it is. Kerlikowske prefers to think of DCIS as a marker of breast cancer risk, not a true precursor. It's not the same as removing polyps during a colonoscopy, which does reduce the incidence of colon cancer, she explains. A colonoscopy can be seen as a preventive measure. Mammography is not. It's not about decreasing the incidence of disease; it's only about finding it.

The NIH panel ended its meeting with a catalogue of research questions aimed at accurate identification of risk for invasive cancer and a better understanding of the biology of DCIS. It also dealt with the psychological impact of diagnosing DCIS as if it were a true cancer. Women who have it "should have access to the best available information and guidance to help make decisions about their care," it urged. The panel's final statement recognized the unwarranted anxiety surrounding a condition with such a low mortality rate. "It is also important," the statement read, "for the medical community to consider eliminating the term 'carcinoma' in this disease, as DCIS is by definition not invasive — a classic hallmark of cancer." It was not within the panel's mandate to make conclusions or recommendations about breast screening, but the panellists agreed that the greatest risk factor for having DCIS is getting a mammogram.

The idea of new nomenclature keeps coming up. DCIS is not the only cancer diagnosis that can lead to overtreatment; it happens with prostate, thyroid, and even lung and skin cancers. In an effort to find solutions to the problem, the NCI called a meeting of experts to assess this overdiagnosis in 2012. After a two-day brainstorming session, the participants decided that their first recommendation was to change cancer terminology. They adopted a new name for non-invasive cancers and precursors: indolent lesion of epithelial origin, or IDLE. *Epithelial* refers to the cells that line the cavities of the body: the stomach, most organs, intestines, esophagus, ducts, and glands. The skin is also made of epithelial cells. The NCI experts agreed that if the medical community learned to see indolent cancers as IDLEs, they'd see them differently and approach them less aggressively. Patients would also be less afraid. A common dictionary defines *idle* as "not active or in use." IDLE might be a fitting acronym to describe something that is not yet cancer or is cancer that is not progressing. But so far, DCIS remains ductal carcinoma in situ.

DCIS continues to present a clinical dilemma. Ten-year survival after treatment for DCIS remains in the 98 percent range. It's estimated that one in every thousand mammograms finds DCIS, making up a quarter of all breast cancers caught by screening. In the United States, it's been calculated that by 2020, one million women will have had a DCIS diagnosis. Although the annual incidence levelled off in the early 2000s, probably due to the rate of mammography screening reaching its maximum point, there are up to sixty thousand new cases each year. The natural history of the condition is still unknown. It's not understood how and when DCIS progresses to invasive cancer. And if it's a precursor to invasive cancer, why don't its detection and surgical removal have a correlating impact on the incidence of invasive cancer? In the absence of answers, lumpectomies with or without radiation or mastectomies remain the medically recommended course. But perhaps not for long: both doctors and patients are advocating for change.

Jan Vick Harris was fifty-five when a routine annual mammogram revealed something suspicious in her breast. A biopsy confirmed cancer, and her radiologist told her she had some options, including a double mastectomy. Although she was devastated and scared, she didn't want a mastectomy and wondered "why on earth" anyone would suggest she have both breasts lopped off. She opted for breast-conserving surgery and radiation, which would begin immediately after the surgery the following week. The surgeon explained that she had DCIS and that it was the least and best cancer she could have, but he intended to treat it aggressively. She had never heard of it. The radiation treatment was new to her too. It was a kind designed to treat internally the specific cancer site in the breast. Known as MammoSite, it involved placing a balloon where the tumour was removed and sewing catheters into the skin. Twice a day, morning and evening for five straight days, Vick Harris subjected herself to having a radiation rod inserted through a catheter into the balloon in her breast.

After the first day, she expressed some reservations about the treatment to her radiologist. She remembers him saying that if she didn't go through with it, she might as well take a loaded gun and aim it at her breast because she was going to lose it. Terrified, she obeyed. Within two weeks of the diagnosis, her radiation treatments were complete, but then she was sent to an oncologist. That's when she learned that the tumour was so small that it had been entirely removed at biopsy. She was completely stunned when the oncologist told her what she had was not cancer and rarely turns into cancer. In a state of disbelief, she asked him to put it in writing. Then she went home to research DCIS.

Vick Harris was diagnosed in 2008. Ten years later, she is well, enjoying retirement after a career in hair dressing and owning a salon, in Chesterfield, South Carolina. But she still worries about the impact of all that radiation, which she would not have consented to had she known then what she knows now. At the time, she was active in a patients' rights group, South Carolina Voices for Patient Safety, which she founded and led following the death of her sister due to a medical error four years earlier. But the feistiness that inspired her to become an advocate for others somehow abandoned her when it was time to look after herself. Even though she had learned to be skeptical and ask questions, she was so fearful of dying and leaving behind her children and grandchildren that she became, she says, incoherent. It clouded her judgment. She's not angry, and she has no quarrel with mammography screening. Her problem is with overtreatment of a non-threatening condition. She also doesn't like being branded as a breast cancer patient because of what it can mean for health insurance. Today, she would take her time, and she is certain that she would opt for a watch-and-wait approach and only accept treatment if invasive cancer developed. She also hopes that her story will embolden others. In 2016, she wrote about her experience and its lesson in an eloquent opinion piece for *JAMA Internal Medicine*. Her plea is that doctors not use fear to encourage patients to comply with a treatment plan and that all patients with DCIS get a range of opinions from different experts and talk to other patients in order to make a considered decision about potentially harmful treatment.

Jan Vick Harris might have liked a conversation with Desiree Basila in San Francisco. Basila is a high-school science teacher but was also doing ballet, and dance was taking up a lot of hours. She hadn't had a mammogram in about seven years. When she was fifty-two, an injury kept her away from the barre, and with time freed up, she thought, *Why not go for a mammogram?* It was June 2007. The mammogram showed an abnormality, which meant that she had to see a surgeon, but she didn't think much of it as others in her family had had cysts. She'll never forget the emotional shock and the incredible animal fear when she got the news. The surgeon walked briskly into the room, snapped the x-ray into the viewer, and said, coldly, yes, it's cancer. It was DCIS. Without giving Basila time to process that information, the surgeon said she was going on holiday in two weeks but had a slot open for a mastectomy. She wanted to perform a biopsy first thing the next morning. Basila, in a panic about having cancer, went for the biopsy. In an examination room, she happened to pick up a booklet about DCIS that had perhaps been forgotten by another patient. She began to read it, took it home, and scoured the internet for more information. After a little research, she said to herself, "Wait a minute. You want me to go in and have my chest chopped off, as a prophylactic measure against getting invasive cancer, and to your knowledge that only happens 20 to 40 percent of the time? That's not going to happen."

With the help of her primary care physician, she wriggled through the rules of her health maintenance organization (HMO) to secure a consultation with another doctor, three months later, in September. That doctor was Shelley Hwang, chief of breast surgery oncology at the University of California, San Francisco, and a leading DCIS researcher.

Basila was seeing the best, and she was hopeful. She had a long list of questions and a lot of ideas about approaches they could take to avoid surgery. Coupled with the extensive research she had done, her background in science made her curious and willing to try different options. But, at first, the meeting did not go well. Basila found Hwang cool and aristocratic. She was a small woman with long dark hair and an amazing posture, carrying herself naturally, not having to work at it. Basila describes her as having an efficient body; it's something that a lithe dancer, also with an aristocratic bearing and her own long, dark, wavy hair, would notice. For her part, Hwang was looking at a woman with a five-centimetre lesion in her breast. Because the mass was large, a lumpectomy would not be good cosmetically, and like the first surgeon, Hwang recommended a mastectomy. Basila persisted with her questions. Hwang kept saying she needed a mastectomy. Disappointed, frustrated, and sensing that Hwang was not happy with the interrogation, Basila decided that the conversation was going nowhere and got up to leave. She plucked her coat from the hook on the door, but just as she was walking out, she turned and asked, "What if I just don't do anything?"

She threw it out there, expecting Hwang to say, "Well, you could do that, but I wouldn't advise it." Then she'd write on Basila's patient record that she'd refused treatment. Instead, Hwang nodded and told her some people were choosing to do that. Basila walked back in and sat down, and suddenly the whole conversation changed. Hwang, she says, just lit up and started talking about her research. She was doing what's called a proof-of-concept trial, where DCIS patients took the drug tamoxifen for three months before undergoing surgery. Basila became part of that trial, but at the end of three months, she still didn't want surgery and dropped out. She continued taking tamoxifen, however, and for a while Hwang saw her every week. She continued to recommend a mastectomy. Basila, the irrepressible science teacher, remained relentless in pushing Hwang, the immovable surgeon, to defy the boundaries and take a chance. After eight months, Basila gave up on tamoxifen because she felt moody and exhausted. Finally, Hwang agreed to active surveillance: every six months, Basila would have an MRI and a mammogram. The term *active surveillance* is considered a better way to describe a watch-and-wait routine, which patients could infer means doing nothing. Basila underwent extensive monitoring. Ten years later, the DCIS remains stable, and she goes for a mammogram just once a year.

As uncomfortable as she was with leaving Desiree Basila's particular DCIS untreated, Hwang was also uncomfortable with growing evidence that many DCIS cases were aggressively overtreated. Like other breast surgeons, she noticed that more women were choosing to have a double mastectomy even though the pre-invasive cells existed in only one breast. Patients believed cutting off the unaffected breast increased the chances of cancer never recurring, or they chose it for cosmetic reasons. When she met Basila in 2007, she and her colleagues were struggling to find the right way to deal with a condition no one understood, worrying about the potential for needless physical and psychological damage to women who would never have come to them were it not for mammography screening. Not that they thought screening was bad, but finding DCIS was an unintended consequence that was now a big problem.

Eventually, Hwang would entertain the possibility of active surveillance as a standard protocol, not just because one stubborn patient and many others demanded it. What she had noticed about double mastectomy rates turned out to be real. In the 1990s, a double mastectomy for DCIS was rare. By 2010, 8 percent of women with the diagnosis chose that course, despite the lack of evidence that this drastic measure made any difference to their survival. In 2011, Hwang moved to North Carolina to become chief of breast surgery at Duke University, where she continued her DCIS research. After some preliminary data showed no difference when women with the most favourable kind of DCIS chose active surveillance, Hwang secured funding for a clinical trial.

The trial, known as COMET (Comparison of Operative to Monitoring and Endocrine Therapy), began recruiting in 2017 and will continue until 2021. Nine hundred women with low-risk DCIS will be randomized to either the standard protocol or to active surveillance and will be followed for two years. In addition to monitoring these women closely to see how many go on to have invasive cancer, the study will collect blood and tissue specimens and do genomic sequencing in the hope of learning how to identify which patients are of such low risk that they can safely opt out of surgery. COMET will also gather information on what it's like to be a DCIS patient, such as how it affects sexuality or impacts financial status. Says Hwang, "This is a very important issue and it's not okay to continue treating patients with very aggressive treatments because we don't know what the alternatives are."

Shelley Hwang's pioneering work earned her a place among *Time* magazine's top one hundred most influential people in the world for 2016, which makes her a rock star in medicine. *Time* co-listed her with another medical rock star, Laura Esserman, also a surgeon and breast cancer oncology specialist and, since 1996, director of the Carol Franc Buck Breast Care Center at the University of California, San Francisco. Media stories about Esserman tend to mention two things: first, she sings to her patients as they are put to sleep in the operating room and even encourages them to send her requests the night before; second, she takes time with her patients, calling them or sending emails to see how they are doing, just about any time of day. She's striking in appearance, in a classy glamorous way, with long blond hair, impeccable clothes, and just the right amount of jewellery. She's also been called a rebel because she's long argued that cancer screening has created a situation where low-risk breast and prostate cancers are overdiagnosed and overtreated. Especially concerned about DCIS, she was an early advocate for active surveillance and as early as 2009 recommended that DCIS be categorized not as cancer but as an IDLE, to classify it as low risk and possibly not needing treatment. "Much of what we call cancer is not destined for an inexorable progression to metastasis and death," she wrote in 2010. "We can no longer say that we must intervene because we cannot tell the difference."

Some of Esserman's research has focused on molecular technology that could help predict the behaviour of indolent lesions to see which ones should be treated. But she also wants to find out how to improve screening by determining who should be screened, at what age, and how often depending on individual risk. Women don't want more screening, she says; they want better screening. One mammogram in ten produces a false positive result. The psychological distress that results is one problem; false positives also make women want to give up on screening. The United States is the only country where it's standard to attend screening beginning at age forty, yet the breast cancer mortality rate is not better than in countries with less screening, Esserman notes. And overdiagnosis is a growing concern. She argues that current screening practices rest on the decades-old assumption that all women have the same risk for the same kind of breast cancer. Insisting that women deserve better than a one-size-fits-all approach, she's launched a massive new study. Her plan is to re-examine screening in light of what we know today: that different breast cancers vary in terms of size, time of onset, rate of growth, and probability of metastasis. Treatments are becoming personalized, so why not personalize screening?

Her study is called the WISDOM trial (Women Informed to Screen Depending on Measures of Risk). It will recruit one hundred thousand women in California between the ages of forty and seventy-four and assign them to either regular screening or individually tailored screening. Regular screening means annual mammograms beginning at age forty. Tailored screening means that the age at which a woman would begin screening, and how often, would depend on risk factors determined by an extensive questionnaire regarding family and health history and a saliva test to look for genetic factors. *BRCA1* and *BRCA2*, the genes linked to hereditary breast and ovarian cancer, are best known, but other, rarer, mutations have also been identified. There are also genetic variants called SNPs (single-nucleotide polymorphisms) or "snips," which are errors along the DNA sequence. There are twenty million SNPs in the human population, and a panel of a hundred or so of them have been implicated in breast cancer risk. Tests for those can provide personal genetic risk scores. The women in the tailored screening group who are at lowest risk will begin screening every two years at age fifty; women at the highest risk will be screened every year beginning at age forty with a breast MRI and a mammogram. In addition to clinical data — rates of cancer, DCIS, false positives, and so on — the study will record how women respond emotionally to screening and its results. A primary goal is to determine whether risk-based screening is as effective for cancer detection as annual screening.

Esserman hopes that the findings from the study will quell the current screening debate. But risk-based screening is in itself contentious. Breast-screening advocates worry that if it leads to fewer people being screened, cancers will be missed because, they argue, in the majority of cases, identifiable risk factors, such as dense breasts or a history in the family, are not present, especially in younger women. Karla Kerlikowske, who for the last several years has focused her research on breast cancer risk, contends that their argument is designed to support annual screening and is not based on current clinical data. She is a principal investigator in the Breast Cancer Surveillance Consortium, a collaboration of mammography registries collecting data on screened women who were found to have breast cancer. A recent research paper found that 90 percent of those women had at least one risk factor. Forty percent of premenopausal and 25 percent of post-menopausal women with breast cancer had dense breasts. Fewer than 10 percent had a family history. Twenty-three percent of post-menopausal women were overweight. Kerlikowske argues that risk factors matter and understanding them will help women avoid what she calls screening failures: missed cancers, interval cancers, and cancers detected only at a late stage. Risk-based screening, rather than age-based screening, might also reduce the rates of overdiagnosis because, says Kerlikowske, as many as thirty percent of women have such low risk they might not ever benefit from screening. The Breast Cancer Surveillance Consortium has developed a consumer-friendly risk calculator accessible on its website.

Esserman's approach to risk-based screening, however, also has critics among screening skeptics. Their concern is that genetic risk scores based on SNPs are low and will scare women without having much impact on mortality, possibly leading to more screening instead of less. In the latter camp, count Steven Narod. He was involved in the analyzed twenty-year data from a national US cancer database called Surveillance, Epidemiology, and End Results, better known as SEER. They looked at close to 110,000 women diagnosed with DCIS from 1988 to 2011 to see how many later died of invasive breast cancer. Three main findings emerged. First, the mortality rate after twenty years was low: only 3.3 percent of women diagnosed with DCIS died of invasive breast cancer. Good news, so far. They also found that regardless of how the women were treated — lumpectomy with radiation, lumpectomy without radiation, or mastectomy — the mortality outcome after twenty years was the same. A few months later, Shelley Hwang's research team would support this important finding in another paper.

The third finding was the "blockbuster," and the one Narod thinks is the most clinically significant. More than half, 54 percent, of the women who died of breast cancer after twenty years did not experience invasive cancer in either breast. In other words, even though the DCIS had not penetrated past the milk ducts and did not result in invasive cancer in the breast, invasive breast cancer showed up elsewhere in the body. Could this mean that the cancer had spread even before the DCIS was removed? It was a stunning observation, and for Narod mind-blowing, raising even more questions than ever about what DCIS really is.

The point of finding DCIS through screening, and treating it, has been to stop a precursor of invasive cancer from plundering healthy tissue. But as Narod wrote in his paper, "If DCIS were truly a non-invasive precursor of breast cancer, then a woman with DCIS should not die of breast cancer without first experiencing an invasive breast cancer" in a breast. "It is often stated that DCIS is a pre-invasive neoplastic lesion that is not lethal in itself," he noted. "The results of the present study suggest this interpretation should be revisited." He suggested that DCIS should be considered to behave no differently than small invasive cancers. Most small invasive cancers don't turn out to be lethally aggressive, but some do. Removing those doesn't mean you've prevented breast cancer death, he says. But proposing that metastasis might have occurred directly on a path from DCIS to some other part of the body, skipping past the steps to invasive cancer in the breast and involvement in the lymph nodes, is a radical idea. Hwang points out that the SEER data Narod looked at have limitations because they don't provide specific information about patients. It's possible that invasive cancer within the breast might have been missed. The theory would need to be tested biologically. It comes back to the need to really understand the natural history of breast cancer.

Then there's a theory that might apply to both DCIS and small invasive cancers. In 2012, Narod wrote a *Current Oncology* editorial provocatively titled "Disappearing Breast Cancers," in which he put forth the argument that a proportion of breast cancers found on mammography, among ones that aren't palpable, will go away on their own. How else to explain, for instance, the drop in invasive cancers so quickly after the HRT scare? If HRT is a cause for new tumours, you would expect that the decline in invasive cancer when HRT is not in the picture would be gradual because it takes time for cancers to grow. The immediate decline, argued Narod, better fits a model in which the removal of estrogen and progesterone leads to the disappearance of an already established cancer. He cited a Swedish study that explained the excess of cancers after six years in a screened group, compared to controls, as likely regression of tumours in the controls. Otherwise, at the end of six years, the number of cancers should have been the same in both groups.

The case of disappearing breast cancer is theoretical and controversial. Narod and others are certain that it happens, but there's no way to know how often or when. The idea that DCIS might metastasize is also theoretical and controversial. But the prevailing wisdom that DCIS is a precursor doesn't answer all the questions either. Narod is focused on figuring out the natural history of breast cancer, suggesting that perhaps all this time we've been chasing the wrong squirrel. "What we think of as cancer, is not cancer," he suggests. "What we're seeing in the breast is only a shadow on the wall and doesn't really predict whether the women will die." This man, who has spent decades in breast cancer research, says, "I'm just learning about it now."

The DCIS research stimulated a curiosity that resulted in a set of theoretical and provocative arguments Narod and his colleague Victoria Sopik developed in *Breast Cancer Research and Treatment* early in 2018. Throwing conventional wisdom aside, they proposed that cancer cells in the breast are not the source of distant metastases and that "if a breast cancer is going to metastasize it will have done so before it is clinically apparent." They proposed that breast cancer does not develop in an orderly, sequential fashion but results from a more dynamic process. Although the hypothesis will seem "out there" to many, it builds on some of the things scientists have wrestled with for decades — for example, how to explain why there is no difference in survival rate whether the surgery choice for DCIS is lumpectomy or mastectomy.

If Narod is right, what could that mean for breast screening? He explains that, yes, the earlier a cancer is identified, the better the survival. But that could be for two reasons. "As cancers get big, they acquire the potential to spread. Or, as cancers get aggressive and spread, they grow faster." The first supports screening; the other doesn't. "We think big cancers are more likely to kill you than small cancers, because cancers that are likely to kill you get big quickly. No one disputes the fact that the larger cancer is the one that kills you. The question is, can I prevent that death by finding a particular cancer when it's smaller?" Bad cancers tend to get big, he says, but that doesn't necessarily imply logically that finding the cancer when it was small can prevent the death.

Narod's opinion is that early detection doesn't work. If screening worked, if stopping DCIS from progressing worked, the number of new invasive breast cancers should go down. But it hasn't, except right after the scare in 2002, when women stopped taking HRT. Screening has led to overdiagnosis and overtreatment not just of DCIS but also of small invasive cancers that are indolent.

Shelley Hwang, Laura Esserman, and Steven Narod are all working at the problems with the early detection paradigm in different ways, but perhaps more important is that all seek a better understanding of how breast cancer works. When is it really cancer? And who will truly benefit from finding it early?

Eleven   LESSONS FROM THE MAMMOGRAM WARS
IN ENGLAND

Breast cancer was a scourge across North America and western Europe in the 1980s, but nowhere was it more lethal than in England, Scotland, and Wales. Every year, breast cancer claimed fifteen thousand lives, one fifth of the total number of cancer deaths among women. The United Kingdom had the highest breast cancer mortality rate in the world. In 1985, the year that the Swedish Two-County trial reported promising results for early detection, Britain's health minister appointed a working group to investigate the implementation of a National Health Service screening program. Patrick Forrest, professor of clinical surgery at the University of Edinburgh and head of an Edinburgh breast screening project, led the group. Forrest had chaired a committee that, just eight weeks before his appointment to the working group was announced, demanded urgent action from the government. That the Forrest group would recommend setting up a public screening service was considered a foregone conclusion.

Forrest laid out a plan to invite all women between the ages of fifty and sixty-four to have mammograms every three years. The government acted quickly and ambitiously. It received the report late in 1986 and only three months later announced that it would have mammography screening in place in some regions by 1988 and nationwide within three years. That was about the time Hazel Thornton, living in the village of Rowhedge, in Colchester, received her letter.

Bending down to pick up the mail from outside her front door one day in August 1991, Thornton was surprised to see an envelope from the National Health Service. It was an invitation to get her breasts screened for cancer, with an appointment for a specific date and time. That's how it's done in England: you're given a precise slot in the schedule. It was the first time she'd ever received such a letter. She was fifty-seven. She and her husband were about to go on a rare holiday to celebrate retirement after the sale of their small irrigation company, but they delayed their vacation so that she could go for her mammogram. She gave it little thought, simply accepting that this was something she should do. "Here was this wonderful health service offering me something, and other women were doing it, so I thought, well, I've got to get one, haven't I?" It would change the course of her life completely.

When she and her husband returned from their holiday in September, another envelope with the results of the mammogram was waiting for her. There was an abnormality. She returned to the clinic promptly, and after being shown the troublesome area on the x-ray, she agreed to have it taken out. Two weeks after the operation, her surgeon told her there was a place for her in a clinical trial. "Well, what have I got?" she asked him. He then mentioned ductal carcinoma in situ, DCIS, and explained that it wasn't full-blown cancer. She'd never heard of DCIS. The surgeon handed her a booklet titled "Living with Breast Surgery," published by the UK Health Education Authority, and said she had two weeks to decide whether she would enter the trial.

Thornton learned from the booklet that the clinical trial was studying four different treatment options: no further treatment, a four- to five-week course of radiation, one tamoxifen tablet daily for five years, or both radiation and tamoxifen. She stared at this, wondering why the treatment options would vary so widely. It must mean, she thought, that doctors had no idea what to do. The leaflet contained little detail about the treatments, and she had little information about her own case. With the help of a friend who worked in the British Medical Association library and another who was a medical student, she immediately set out to research this thing called DCIS. She turned up some papers suggesting that the serious side effects of radiotherapy couldn't be justified. That convinced her. She had no interest in being part of a trial where she could end up receiving radiation therapy. But she was stunned that she was being asked to decide so quickly, with so little to go on. She thought entrance into a clinical trial was supposed to be based on informed consent. This was not anything like informed consent in her view, and she was appalled. Equipped with the organizational prowess, attention to detail, and stubbornness she had learned to harness in order to survive as an independent businesswoman, she segued seamlessly into activism.

She couldn't stop thinking about the clinical trial, and she couldn't stop researching. One morning at half past five, she shot up in bed. "I've got it," she said to herself and grabbed a pencil to write a letter to her surgeon explaining why she couldn't be involved. She wasn't even sure he'd have time to read it. But he responded quickly. He thought her letter was so cogent that he forwarded it to Michael Baum, an eminent breast surgeon. Baum wrote to Thornton asking to meet. Meanwhile, she began to think there must be hundreds of women like her up and down the country, so she fired off what she'd written to several journals. She had to go to the library and look up which ones might be most likely to be interested. All of this happened before Christmas, within a few short months of her surgery. The *Lancet* was the first to accept her article and published it on January 4, 1992. Thornton was not a medical researcher, had no university education, and had never seen a copy of the *Lancet*, but the editors were impressed with the eloquence of her arguments. Former staff member Imogen Evans remembers immediately handing the article to her boss because it was such a breath of fresh air. When Evans called to say the *Lancet* would like to publish the article, the silence on the other end of line lasted for a good thirty seconds. Thornton couldn't believe what she was hearing.

The article was titled "Breast Cancer Trials: A Patient's Viewpoint." In it, Thornton described the research journey that resulted in her decision to forego the DCIS trial. "A woman is given a diagnosis that she has never heard of before and a leaflet indicating four widely differing treatment options," she wrote. "She has two weeks to deliberate and seek further information. This scenario begs the question: what is informed consent?" Thornton suggested that such a request makes a woman feel isolated at a time when she needs support, when she expects a treatment plan but instead is sent off to make a decision on her own, deprived of proper consultation with her surgeon. "To ask your average woman-in-the-street to have to decide whether to take part, in the moment she has just been told she has a carcinoma, would seem to be asking just too much." It was a beautifully reasoned piece in an important journal, and now she was a published author.

Thornton's big sky-blue eyes twinkle with merriment and a hint of mischief as she describes how she's always "just got on." She giggles a little over her success as a champion for patients' rights, as if surprised by the recognition her work has earned. She simply fell into it, and one thing led to another: articles in medical journals, countless speaking engagements, a book, an honorary doctorate. Now eighty-three years old, she still checks the *BMJ* website on a daily basis to keep tabs on things. And she still gets angry at "beastly closed-minded" people she has "no truck with." Her self-deprecating reflections on her achievements, mixed with a sense of humour, disguise a tough and determined mind. So does her diminutive size. She walks steadily, leading the way up a flight of stairs in London's British Library and showing off the architecture at St. Pancras Station, but she is ethereally thin, as though she might evaporate. Beneath a blue plaid cap, wisps of white hair sneak out and delicately frame a pixie-like face. The cap, called a baker boy hat in England, is made of Welsh lamb's wool and is light and comfortable enough to wear all day, with a brim over her forehead to shield her sensitive eyes from glare. If she is exhausted by a two-hour train trip from her rural home, she doesn't show it. A small bowl of soup with some bread suffices for lunch.

Her success with the *Lancet* inspired her to send articles to other journals, and things escalated. She launched into her accidental advocacy curious and driven. With the help of a medical dictionary and scientist friends, she schooled herself in the numeracy of studies and learned to navigate the jargon of medical literature. She became a scholar. She's written more than two hundred papers and commentaries of her own and has also been a reviewer. She jokes that as a reviewer, she irons out some of the language. "I bring a bit of a human touch to it," she says. "Sociological talk can be convoluted." In 1995, Michael Baum asked her to chair the Consumers Advisory Group for Clinical Trials he was establishing, and she threw herself into that for five years, becoming the authoritative voice on involving patient input in research. Since 2001, she has been an honorary visiting fellow in the Department of Epidemiology and Public Health at the University of Leicester. In 2002, the university granted her an honorary doctorate of science for her contribution to medicine and patient care. The press release described her as "fearless" and "trail blazing." In 2006, she co-authored a book, *Testing Treatments*, with Imogen Evans (who had left the *Lancet* to work at the Medical Research Council); Iain Chalmers, founder of the Cochrane Collaboration; and Paul Glaszniou, then director of evidence-based medicine at Oxford.

Wanting to change the rules around clinical trials was the starting point, but patient advocacy led Thornton to look critically at other areas of medicine, including early detection of breast cancer. She wrote prolifically about screening issues and became one of the biggest critics of the UK breast screening program. Michael Baum, considered one of England's leading breast surgeons and breast cancer researchers, was right alongside her.

Michael Baum can count a long list of accomplishments in cancer research and leadership. He was appointed professor of surgery at King's College medical school in 1980, where he began to specialize in treating breast cancer. At the same time, he obtained funding for the Cancer Research Campaign Clinical Trials Centre and became its director. Baum's research group was the first to show that the drug tamoxifen increased breast cancer survival; he was a principal investigator in a huge international cancer trial comparing tamoxifen to another treatment (anastrozole). At the clinical trials centre, his group developed ethical models for randomized trials and for informed consent procedures, and his work has been celebrated internationally with many awards. He's a giant in medicine. Now in his eighties, and although small in physical stature, he is sturdy and robust, with square-jawed intensity and purpose. When he explains how he came to be a breast-screening dissenter, his tone is genuine concern layered with sadness.

Baum hadn't been involved in any breast screening initiatives, and he had no input in the Forrest report. But when the government adopted its recommendations, he got "sucked in," as he describes it: he and the head of radiology at King's College Hospital were instructed to establish a screening centre for southeast London and have it open within twelve months. It would be one of the first in the country, and it would also serve as one of a handful of training centres for radiologists. They worked day and night to get the centre started, while at the same time doing their regular jobs. He visited screening centres in Europe to see how they were doing things, and the model he liked best was one in Holland, set up in a shopping centre. So they picked a spot on a little street called Butterfly Walk, in a shopping centre not far from the hospital. Baum did all of this in good faith, and he enjoyed the status and prestige that came with it. But before long, he was seeing things he found disturbing.

As a surgeon, he saw the women who came out on the other side of screening, the ones who needed further tests because the mammograms found something suspicious. He worried about what he called "the hordes of worried well" flooding breast clinics and clogging up resources better dedicated to those genuinely in need of diagnosis and treatment. In an introduction to a 1990 report on breast cancer services in London, he said clinics like his at King's College hadn't been given money to deal with the extra work; it was just assumed that existing services would absorb the expanded demand. He also worried that screening was causing needless anxiety and harm. "In terms of false lumps, unnecessary biopsies, unnecessary cancer labels being attached to patients and the difficulty in getting life insurance, as well as the unnecessary mastectomies in borderline cases, I suspect the balance has gone the other way and the costs to women are increasing rather than decreasing," he wrote. Among patients referred to his clinic, the ratio of benign to malignant cases had doubled since the beginning of screening.

Among the things that first bothered him was the issue of informed consent — or rather the lack of it — in the way women were invited to screening. Giving them a specific appointment, on a certain date, at a certain time, was a summons, not an invitation, he felt, and women would assume that it was mandatory. If they didn't comply, they received stern reminders. He thought women were pressured into the program and not told about the limitations or drawbacks or the issue of finding DCIS. He remembers that a woman diagnosed with DCIS was one of his first surgical patients after the introduction of screening. His consultation with the woman went something like this: "The good news is we caught it early. So your mastectomy is booked in two weeks." The woman replied, "But you've said it's early; why am I having the mastectomy?" It's an exaggeration of the conversation, Baum admits, but it was a real scenario, and the patient was devastated. As the years went on, he became more and more distressed realizing what a terrible thing it is to do a mastectomy for early breast cancer. The false positives generated in screening and the resulting anxiety also distressed him.

Baum moved from King's College, and its breast-screening centre, to be a professor of surgery at the Royal Marsden Hospital and Institute of Cancer Research in 1990. But he remained a member of the national advisory committee to the National Health Service breast screening program, and by this time, screening centres had opened across the United Kingdom. As additional information from screening trials came in — by 1992, there were six — it was becoming clear to him that the estimates of benefit were becoming narrower, whereas the estimates of harm were getting wider. His doubts about screening deepened when, in 1995, the *Lancet* published an article co-authored by Charles Wright, the Canadian surgeon. Wright and fellow surgeon C. Barber Mueller looked at all the trials and concluded that the number of women screened to save one life per year ranged from 7,086 in the most promising trial to 63,264 in the least. The benefit was minimal at best. Then they calculated the cost per life saved. Adding the cost of further tests because of false positives to the cost of lost work, travel, and after-care for patients, the total could exceed a million dollars. Balancing the benefits against the harms and the financial costs, they concluded that public funding for breast screening was not justifiable. Michael Baum responded to this provocative *Lancet* article with a letter to the editor titled "Screening for Breast Cancer, Time to Think — and Stop?" He wrote that it is, of course, invidious to put a price tag on a woman's life but asked if the large sum of money could be redirected in services and research "in such a way that more women would benefit and fewer well women would be harmed." He argued that the screening clinics should be turned into specialist clinics to serve women with symptoms and funding for clinical trials of new therapies would be more cost-effective.

Baum was still a member of the national advisory committee to the screening program, but not for much longer. At an emergency meeting called to deal with unfavourable reports about screening, he spoke out. He questioned what the UK program was telling women. He wanted leaflets that outlined fairly all the harms as well as the benefits, and instead of using the vague relative percentage of lives saved, he wanted absolute numbers that would be clear about exactly how many lives that would be. The leaflets told women that screening would reduce mortality by 25 percent. Baum wanted women to understand that it was 25 percent of a small number, and he wanted the invitations to be specific about how many women needed to be screened over ten years to save one life. He recalls clearly what the chair of the committee said: "But Professor Baum, if we did that the women wouldn't come." The program's target was to have 70 percent of eligible women participate. So far, it was reaching that goal, but anything reflecting negatively on the idea of early detection might make the numbers go down. Baum thought hoarding information was completely unethical, and in 1997, he resigned.

Baum saw himself as someone with a different perspective than the public health people and radiologists who were fervent about screening.

He was working at the "sharp end"; as a surgeon, he picked up the pieces. He also had a different perspective on the natural history of disease. The conventional wisdom, as succinctly spelled out in the Forrest report, was that breast cancer starts in the milk-producing cells of the breast and the cells lining the milk ducts. At first, the cancer is confined within the milk ducts, but as it grows, it invades surrounding tissue and then spreads to lymph nodes before finally metastasizing in another part of the body, such as the bone, liver, or brain. This was the basic premise behind early detection: catch it early and stop it before it spreads.

Some of the DCIS cases Baum encountered made him skeptical. The breast is considered to have four quadrants, and a cancer that appears in more than one of those quadrants is multifocal. When DCIS is multifocal, a mastectomy is standard because it's all over the breast. If DCIS is just one well-defined lump, a simple lumpectomy suffices to remove the offending tissue. At least half of Baum's DCIS cases in the early 1990s were multifocal, yet an invasive cancer that is multifocal is very rare, suggesting that assumptions about how breast cancer developed might be wrong. Baum picks up a pen and notebook and draws a graph to illustrate another important observation. He draws a steep upward curve representing a steady rise in DCIS since the advent of screening. He draws a steep downward curve that intersects with the first to show how the incidence of invasive cancer should have gone down because of all the cancers supposedly caught early. But that's not what's happened. The incidence of invasive cancer is a steady flat line. Screening has had no impact on the rate of invasive cancer. The theory doesn't hold. From the very early days of screening, Michael Baum saw that what was thought to be the natural course of breast cancer might be wrong. He's since proposed a theory, based on what's known in mathematics as chaos theory, that for DCIS to progress to invasive cancer requires a collision of coincidental circumstances that tip the balance at a specific moment. Baum suggests that those triggering circumstances could depend on unpredictable changes within the precancerous cells combined with something else going on the host body, much as the slightest changes can cause complex weather systems to shift. The difference is that mathematicians have figured out how to predict those shifts and forecast whether or not it will be rainy or windy. Doctors have no way to predict when DCIS will cross the threshold to invasive cancer.

As Hazel Thornton broadened her research, she, too, began to have questions about the rationale for screening. She had started out wanting to change the way patients were recruited into clinical trials, but then she began to ask herself why she was so willing to submit to the government's invitation to the breast-screening clinic in the first place. She had believed it was a good thing, but on what basis? She realized that the information she'd received was inadequate and imbalanced. The leaflet sent to her said, "If the disease is discovered early enough, there is a very good chance of making a full recovery." There was no hint that the mammogram would find asymptomatic lesions such as DCIS, where it wasn't at all clear what should be done. There was no hint of uncertainty. She had learned that one in every five women diagnosed with breast cancer because of screening had DCIS, and most of those women would not go on to have invasive cancer. Why wasn't that information provided in the screening invitation? Thornton's view was that women were summoned to take part in a dubious preventive measure, imposed upon the public without proper debate or understanding. She and Michael Baum joined forces in a fight to get more balanced content into the leaflets. They both describe exasperating, endless correspondence with Julietta Patnick, director of the National Health Service breast screening program in England, and say that getting anything to change was a slow process. Patnick also remembers the to and fro. She says each time a change was made, new complaints would surface. It would take the work of a young researcher at the Nordic Cochrane Centre in Denmark to bring the simmering controversy to a public boil.

Karsten Jørgensen was a medical student when he heard Peter Gøtzsche lecture on the systematic reviews of medical literature. Jørgensen, who hadn't yet settled on a specialty, was fascinated when Gøtzsche described how the pharmaceutical industry could manipulate clinical trials and explained the importance of doctors having information about drugs from independent analyses of trial data. Jørgensen became smitten with the idea of doing the kind of research that Gøtzsche was talking about and began working with the Nordic Cochrane Centre in 2002. Wanting to follow up on his controversial review of breast cancer screening published in the *Lancet* in 2001, Gøtzsche gave Jørgensen an assignment. He asked him to look at websites to see what health authorities or patients' groups were saying about mammography screening and compare that information to the findings of the Cochrane breast-screening review. Were any harms of screening mentioned? What kind of numbers did they use? Were benefits or harms expressed in relative percentage terms, or were they expressed in absolute terms so that the numbers of individuals benefited or harmed were clear? Would it be possible to look at the material and compare benefits to harms?

Jørgensen is now the deputy director of the Nordic Cochrane Centre and has produced numerous reviews and research papers for an array of the world's most important journals, engaging in greatly more complicated work than that first easy assignment. The centre is in a modern low-rise building of concrete and glass on the outskirts of central Copenhagen, and Jørgensen's office is spacious and bright, even though the sky is grey. He's casually neat in a sweater and jeans — lean, tall, and clean-cut with brown hair cut close to the scalp. His surroundings are equally organized; there is none of the clutter you might expect from a scientist who spends long hours buried in reams of data. He's down to earth and personable, and it's evident that he loves his work. The rookie assignment researching websites had an indelible effect. "What I didn't know at the time," he says, "is that research doesn't have to be difficult to do in order to be important. What's equally important is the question you raise, the question at the edge of where science is, and is it something that matters to people?" It was a valuable lesson. The research also made him angry — angry about how the way information is selected and presented can manipulate thinking. On those two different levels, a revelation got him started on years of investigation into mammography screening.

Jørgensen looked at the websites of thirteen organizations he labelled as advocacy groups, such as the American Cancer Society and the Canadian Cancer Society. He also looked at the websites of eleven government institutions (such as BreastScreen Australia and the National Health Service Breast Screening Programme) and three consumer groups (such as the US National Breast Cancer Coalition) in English-speaking and Scandinavian countries. He found that advocacy groups and government agencies provided poor information severely biased in favour of screening. The consumer groups offered more balanced and more comprehensive information. When he completed his paper, Gøtzsche said they should submit it to the *BMJ*. Jørgensen thought the *BMJ* wouldn't consider it important enough, but he was wrong. The journal published the article on January 17, 2004.

"It is worrying," Jørgensen wrote, "that so few websites live up to accepted standards of informed consent." He argued that the way information is presented affects choices. For example, a leaflet that asks, "Why do I need breast screening?" sends a different message than one headed "Do I need breast screening?" The websites he examined most commonly said, based on a review of Swedish data, that screening reduces mortality in women aged fifty to sixty-nine by 30 percent, without saying anything about the actual number of deaths or lives saved. Jørgensen wrote that the same data would mean that screening one thousand women over ten years would result in one life saved from breast cancer death. The absolute risk of dying of breast cancer would be reduced by 0.1 percent. Jørgensen found that although the majority of websites exaggerated the benefits of screening, they underestimated or ignored the harms. "It is inappropriate," he wrote, "to continue to use information purely for encouraging high uptake."

The next step was to look at screening invitations. Jørgensen collected invitations from thirty-one screening programs in the United Kingdom, Canada, Australia, Denmark, New Zealand, Norway, and Sweden. Again, he found a heavy bias in favour of screening, with exaggeration of benefit and no mention of overdiagnosis and overtreatment. His analysis in the *BMJ* in 2006 argued that because screening programs need women to participate, they are in a conflict of interest if they are also responsible for dispensing the information. And when information is not balanced, informed consent is distorted. Jørgensen finds this especially reprehensible as the women invited to screening are not patients seeking help for a specific problem but healthy people who are approached by a health authority and told what to do in a situation where the option of not attending screening is a reasonable choice.

In that 2006 paper, Jørgensen outlined what he and Gøtzsche thought a properly balanced invitation should contain. They assumed a 15 percent reduction in breast cancer mortality and an overdiagnosis rate of 30 percent, based on the most recent Cochrane analysis of the randomized trials. If two thousand women are screened for ten years, one will avoid dying from breast cancer. With screening, 1,800 women will be alive; without screening, 1,799 will be alive. Among two thousand women screened, ten healthy women will be treated unnecessarily. Four of those ten will have a breast removed, whereas six will receive breast-conserving surgery and most likely radiation therapy.

Three years later, the Nordic Cochrane Centre went at the issue again in the *BMJ*, this time focusing solely on the National Health Service breast screening leaflet *Breast Screening: The Facts*, written in 2002 and revised in 2006. Peter Gøtzsche had become impatient. In an article bluntly titled "Breast Screening: The Facts — or Maybe Not," he criticized the leaflet for telling English women only that screening would save fourteen hundred lives each year, without mentioning that ten times more women risked being overdiagnosed and treated for a disease they did not have. The leaflet made no mention of DCIS. Gøtzsche suggested that the leaflet violated a rule established by the General Medical Council, a UK oversight body: "You must tell patients if an investigation or treatment might result in a serious adverse outcome, even if the likelihood is very small." He put forward a template for a new leaflet.

Gøtzsche had consulted Hazel Thornton and Michael Baum, who had been lobbying for better information all along. They followed up his article with an angry letter to the editor of the *Times*, published on February 19, 2009. Baum's signature led those of twenty-two other cancer experts, epidemiologists, family doctors, and patient representatives, Thornton among them. In the flurry of media that erupted, Baum told a medical reporter it was imperative that the leaflet be rewritten. "None of the invitations for screening comes close to telling the truth," he stated. Within days, England's national cancer director announced that a formal review was in progress and a new leaflet would likely be ready by fall.

The movement gained momentum as more voices rallied for change. Iona Heath was elected president of the Royal College of General Practitioners in June 2009, the same month that she published a gloves-off opinion piece in the *BMJ*. Angry that the breast screening leaflet mentioned only benefits, she declared that she, herself, had "cheerfully declined" any invitations to go for a mammogram but worried that the information on which she based that decision was not made available to her patients. Hers was an individual decision, and other women with a different perception of their risk will appropriately make a different decision, she wrote. "It is not wrong to say yes," she concluded, "but neither is it wrong to say no."

Heath wrote that *BMJ* piece after decades of experience as a general practitioner made her increasingly concerned about a medical-industrial complex pushing diagnostic criteria closer and closer to normal to get more and more people into treatment. For instance, we no longer have just diabetes, we have prediabetes. The threshold for treating people for high blood pressure has lowered. Heath is now retired from practice but remains active in the debate around overdiagnosis and overtreatment and is an advocate for "less is more" in medicine. In the cozy environs of her well-worn living room, she is reflective and philosophical. As she speaks, she sprinkles quotations from this and that author to illustrate her points, just as she does in the many essays she's written. She is soft-spoken and thoughtful. Her approach is at once intellectual, as a writer who must think things through, and practical, as a person who's guided patients through worry, ill health, and sometimes death.

Seeing how patients suffered made Heath skeptical about early diagnosis. "You see how frightened and worried people become by a diagnosis when they are basically well," she explains. "You see a shadow crossing their lives." She worries that people become conscious of their health in a way that is not conducive to health. She describes women in a full-blown state of anxiety because they were recalled after a mammogram. Heath also noticed that after the breast-screening program became established, she seemed to see more of her patients doing very well long after their breast cancer diagnoses. Although on the surface this was good news, she wondered how many were overdiagnosed, their lives unnecessarily blighted.

A doctor who says publicly she forgoes screening sends a strong message. But in her office, when patients asked for her advice, she didn't try to persuade them to take the same course. Instead, she discussed the information in Gøtzsche's proposed leaflet. The opportunity for discussion didn't come up often, however, because in England, women receive the invitations to screening directly. And if a patient came to her after being told she had breast cancer, Heath could never tell her she might have been overdiagnosed. For one thing, there was no way to know for certain. For another, the patient had a different narrative. As far as she was concerned, her life had been saved. Iona Heath articulated all of this in her eloquent plea that women be given the truth about the damage early detection can do. But the fall of 2009 came and went without the promised new leaflet.

Meanwhile, the pro-screening lobby was attacking the *BMJ* for a lack of balance in its content on screening. Managing editor Fiona Godlee wanted to address that concern, but she found that articles offered from the screening side and sent out for peer review were not well argued. As the journal published more on the controversy and the critics became more vocal, Godlee decided to find an independent voice to look at what the *BMJ* had published and at the evidence in favour of screening. She approached Klim McPherson, an epidemiologist at Oxford University. The *BMJ* published his review in June 2010. Unexpectedly, McPherson's conclusions were less favourable to screening than anything the journal had published before. The review was a condemnation.

McPherson put forward a new set of numbers showing that the difference screening was making to mortality was very small. In 2009, the US Preventive Services Task Force concluded that, based on data from all of the screening trials, mammography screening reduced mortality by 15 percent. In the United Kingdom, the breast cancer mortality rate was 0.41 percent in women aged forty to fifty-five, and at age sixty, the risk of death over the next fifteen years was 1.2 percent. Women are rarely told the risk of death is that low, and as McPherson pointed out, it's not well understood that reducing such a low mortality rate by 15 or even 30 percent is a minimal return. The reason it is not understood, he wrote, is "obfuscation from organizers of mammography services assuming that a positive emphasis is needed to ensure reasonable compliance." Using the same kind of absolute numbers for overdiagnosis, McPherson found that the individual risk of overdiagnosis due to screening, although difficult to estimate, was also very low, but certainly there was harm. One in every five screened detected cancers was DCIS, and the uncertainty of what to do with this diagnosis was a dilemma. In a sharply worded conclusion, McPherson said a misplaced propaganda battle and arguments that polarize were unhelpful; for too long, women had been misled and confused. He wondered how the breast screening program could exist with so many unanswered questions and called for a full examination of all the data.

The promised new leaflet was finally published on December 13, 2010, a year later than promised and more than a decade after people such as Michael Baum and Hazel Thornton first demanded that women receive accurate information. Julietta Patnick, the screening program's director, explained that the leaflet was the result of a long process of reviewing the randomized trials and the UK data and then "rigorously testing" a draft in focus groups. Then "clinical and language experts" vetted it "to ensure accuracy and clarity." But far from quelling the controversy, the new leaflet created more.

The leaflet stated that for every four hundred women screened for ten years, one fewer would die from breast cancer. Peter Gøtzsche was astounded. "There is no way this could be claimed," he said. Such a figure, three times higher than the most optimistic estimates from the trials and five times higher than modern estimates, was "outrageous." An equally livid Michael Baum agreed. "The agents of the state are behaving in an almost Stalinist fashion to coerce women into an activity that has marginal benefit," he said. The leaflet alluded to the harms of screening but did not quantify them. "Sometimes a mammogram will not look normal and you will be recalled for more tests, but cancer is not there," the leaflet read. "This is called a false positive result." It also skirted the issue of overdiagnosis: "Screening can find cancers which are treated but which may not otherwise have been found during your lifetime." Gøtzsche found this wording manipulative and said a woman would probably think, *Great. That's why I go for screening, to find cancers that wouldn't otherwise be found.*

The chair of the breast screening program's advisory committee, epidemiologist Valerie Beral from the University of Oxford, defended the estimate of mortality reduction — one fewer death for every four hundred women screened — saying it derived from a review the committee undertook in 2006. Deaths from breast cancer had been reduced by half since the advent of screening, she said, although she acknowledged that much of this decline was due not to screening but to treatment. As for the vagueness in the information about harms, she declared that women in the focus groups said they didn't want statistics.

Susan Bewley might argue with that. Bewley, a professor of obstetrics at King's College London, was approaching fifty and, with a family history of breast cancer, was considering whether to accept an invitation to screening. She declined because, after looking at the evidence, she saw that the National Health Service was not telling the whole truth. Bewley, an occasional contributor to the *BMJ*, told editor Fiona Godlee that she'd written to Mike Richards. Richards was England's cancer czar, the national clinical director for cancer and end-of-life care at the National Health Service. She'd asked him why the breast screening information wasn't more balanced, but she didn't get much of an answer. Richards told her that many experts in the United Kingdom didn't agree with the Nordic Cochrane Centre's methodology. Godlee had an idea. She suggested that Bewley write an open letter to Richards and tell him the *BMJ* would publish it and his response, side by side. Bewley crafted a persuasive argument that evidence-based medicine replace "eminence-based medicine." Even if many experts in the United Kingdom disagreed with Cochrane, she wrote, women had a right to be told there was much uncertainty about the benefits of early detection and, in fact, those benefits were marginal at best. She joined the call for an independent review, "a real, unbiased review that would not be kicked into the long grass, whose findings would be widely and properly disseminated." The letters appeared in print on October 25, 2011. Richards's response signalled that, finally, things might change. He announced the initiation of an independent review. There would be a new process to develop the written information all cancer screening programs provided to the public, and the breast-screening leaflet would be the first revised.

Richards asked Michael Marmot, an epidemiologist at University College London, to conduct the review. Marmot assembled a panel of experts in medical statistics or breast cancer who had never published any work on breast screening. The panel revisited independent reviews from Denmark, the United States, and Canada; sifted through the studies; and listened to expert testimony. The focus was on mortality and overdiagnosis in the UK context. Marmot's report, made public in October 2012, at long last gave women a more realistic idea of what the breast screening program could do for them. It estimated that for every ten thousand women who participated in screening for twenty years, forty-three breast cancer deaths would be prevented and 129 cases of breast cancer would be overdiagnosed. For every woman whose life was saved, three would endure unnecessary surgery and possibly treatment. With the caveat that the estimates were uncertain, the panel concluded that the breast screening program should continue, but clear information about the harms and benefits was essential in a modern health care system.

This was hardly the end of the story. Both sides in the screening debate disputed the findings. Baum and Gøtzsche both argued that the Marmot panel overestimated the number of lives that would be saved and underestimated the frequency of overdiagnosis. They thought the harms of overdiagnosis, the toxic effects of radiation and chemotherapy that could even be fatal, were underplayed. Baum argued that radiation therapy increases the risk of ischemic heart disease and lung cancer, and the number of deaths from those causes could surpass the number of lives saved. Others thought the rate of overdiagnosis among screened women was exaggerated. Marmot estimated that it was 19 percent. Stephen Duffy, a London epidemiologist who worked with László Tabár, argued in the *Lancet* that the true figure was likely a quarter of that. But the report was an important step in its clear recognition that early detection was not what screening proponents represented, a step away from the paternalism that kept women from hearing the truth and toward meaningful informed consent.

Today in England, the invitation to screening is a thirteen-page leaflet that provides information about both benefits and harms using absolute numbers. Gone is the promise that screening reduces deaths by 25 percent, a relative number that can be very misleading. Instead, women are told that every year in the United Kingdom, about thirteen hundred lives are saved, whereas four thousand cancers are overdiagnosed. Those numbers are from the Marmot report. Screening critics would say they still exaggerate the benefit and fail to account for lives saved because of better treatments rather than screening. Baum thinks it's a falsehood to say screening saves any lives, but both he and Hazel Thornton agree that, although not perfect, the leaflet is a considerable improvement. Its tone is neutral, with these opening words: "It is your choice whether to have breast screening or not. This leaflet aims to help you decide." It explains DCIS.

What's underscored in this whole long fight in the United Kingdom is the inevitable flaw of many screening programs. The National Health Service implemented breast screening with the best of intentions, when women were dying of breast cancer at an alarming rate. But in order for screening to make a difference to those horrible mortality statistics, at least 70 percent of women had to participate. So what message do you send out? Obviously, an encouraging one, or else you won't get the numbers. Meanwhile, an institution becomes entrenched, hard to steer in a different direction even when it's apparent that better treatment might have more impact on mortality than mammograms and the harms of overdiagnosis must be recognized. It's a lesson not lost on Fiona Godlee, who has for many years steered the *BMJ* in a campaign against "too much medicine." Medicine is often based on problematic evidence, she says, giving a lot of scope for people to push their own agendas, their own enthusiasms. Patient groups and relatives of people who've died of cancer bring a lot of emotion that overlies "a rather crummy evidence base." There are a lot of vested interests because it's cancer.

Godlee has been editor-in-chief of the *BMJ* since 2005 and is the first woman to hold that position. She is tall, with blond, wavy, bobbed hair and wholesome apple cheeks. She is fifty-six — screening age. So far, she has turned down the invitations to screening and has said so publicly in speeches. She once held the view that if you were moderately informed, you could have your breast screening, and you could be told you've got something. Then you could have the conversation, and you could decide not to do anything about it. But Michael Baum made her think about it again, and she's come to realize that screen-detected cancer and symptom-detected cancer are different. "If you end up finding a lump then that's a different matter than if you have a lump detected from screening." Susan Bewley and Iona Heath also had an impact on her thinking. Godlee has an influential position, and her height makes her imposing physically too. But she has no air of arrogance or superiority, and as she recounts the steps on the way to the Marmot report, she is friendly and open in describing the considerations that went into the journal's approach. For the *BMJ*, it was a victory. Godlee says, however, it's important to always keep in mind the evidence of the moment. Medicine should evolve with new information. She is aware that being public about her own decision to forgo screening could influence other women, but she's not saying she's forever against the idea of screening. If new evidence shifted the equation between benefit and harm, she would reconsider her choice.

Twelve KEPT IN THE DARK

England's breast screening program is not the only one guilty of incomplete and misleading information. Take, for example, what women in Ontario are told. "I am writing to ask you to get screened for breast cancer," begins the letter from Linda Rabeneck, vice-president of prevention and cancer control at Cancer Care Ontario. "The best way to protect your health is by getting a mammogram every two years." On the back of the one-page letter is a list of "facts" that includes the statements "most women will have normal mammogram results" and "regular mammograms are the best way for women ages fifty to seventy-four to reduce the risk of dying of breast cancer." The letter provides instructions on how to book an appointment.

With the letter comes a small pamphlet with colour photos of women getting mammograms. The women look young, with a few years to go before their fiftieth birthday. Screening can reduce deaths from breast cancer, the pamphlet promises, because with early detection, "there is a better chance of treating the cancer successfully." Acknowledging the imperfections in screening, the pamphlet does say mammography might miss some cancers. It also advises that some detected lesions may never cause symptoms, and some women might have surgery or treatment for breast cancer that isn't life threatening.

But overall, the information is scant and vague and leans heavily toward the benefits of screening. The pamphlet tells us that every year in Ontario, nine thousand women will be diagnosed with breast cancer, and 1,980 will die. Without context, those numbers look terrifying.

The truth is that deaths from breast cancer account for just 14 percent of all cancer deaths among women and add up to half the number of deaths from lung cancer. Fewer than 3 percent of women in Canada or the United States will die from breast cancer. The pamphlet offers no actual numbers on how many lives early detection might save or how often indolent cancers are overdiagnosed. The problem of false positives — where a mammogram looks suspicious but a biopsy reveals no cancer — isn't even mentioned.

In its pat-on-the-head tone that implies "just trust me, I know what's good for you," the personalized letter from Cancer Care Ontario avoids details. The "facts" as outlined aren't precise enough to give a true picture, and the letter's simple message that "the best way to protect your health is by getting a mammogram every two years" exaggerates. The language almost suggests that a mammogram will prevent cancer, even though all it can do is find it, and not all of the time. The letter implies that a mammogram trumps all other health protection measures a woman might take, ranging from vaccinations to balanced diets to exercise. The final page of the pamphlet does note that a healthy lifestyle might reduce the risk of breast cancer, but "most importantly, get screened," it says. The pamphlet directs women to a website that provides no detailed information about the risks and benefits of mammograms — only another simple pitch, in twenty-eight languages, that early detection saves lives.

Every Canadian province has its own screening program with its own guidelines, and the depth of information provided to women varies but typically is as vague as the information provided in Ontario. Some provinces quantify the mortality benefit of screening, and the estimate ranges from 15 to 25 percent in one to 25 to 35 percent in another. Some websites mention the possibility of overdiagnosis without providing any estimate of how often it happens. In general, screening programs are more focused on getting as many people to participate as possible than on giving good-quality, unbiased information.

Quebec is the exception. In contrast to others, the Quebec program attempts to lay out specific and detailed information. Its stated goal is to reduce breast cancer deaths by 25 percent, but note that it's a goal, not presented as fact. A program brochure tells women that for every one thousand women in Quebec who take part in screening for twenty years, it's estimated that thirteen will die of breast cancer regardless, compared to twenty who will die if they don't get screened. Over a twenty-year screening period, nearly half of women will be called back for at least one additional test, resulting in waiting and worrying. Seventy-seven cancers will be diagnosed; twenty-one of them will be interval cancers, detected between the routine screens. Ten of the seventy-seven will be overdiagnosed; the cancers would not progress to cause any harm if undetected. Only in Quebec is the problem of overdiagnosis quantified in this way. "It's your decision," the brochure states. "The decision will depend on what is important for you and on your values." Compared to the language of insistent urgency in Ontario, the language is neutral. Quebec's program comes closer to what can be found on the Nordic Cochrane Centre website, where an updated version of the pamphlet initially written for the United Kingdom is available in many languages. It is a highly readable twelve pages outlining the pros and cons of breast screening in detail, complete with a list of sources.

Breast screening programs have a mandate to bring women in, but some breast cancer charities are also complicit in suppressing information. Perhaps the most egregious example of misleading messaging was the Canadian Breast Cancer Foundation's GOHAVE1 campaign. The charity's British Columbia/Yukon branch launched the campaign in 2005 with a million-dollar grant from the provincial government. Campaign literature directed women to a phone number — 1-844-GOHAVE1 — that connected callers to the provincial screening program to book an appointment quickly. The foundation produced a memorable little video that became the campaign's core message. In the video, a woman peels what appears to be a smallish navel orange and lets it sit in the palm of her hand. We're told the orange represents the possible size of a lump that a woman might feel in her breast. She eats, takes a pit out of her mouth, and holds the tiny seed between two fingers. This is said to be the possible size of a lump visible on a mammogram. In the campaign the following year, during breast cancer month in October, volunteers wearing orange T-shirts were dispatched to grocery stores to hand out fresh oranges along with GOHAVE1 educational material.

Other regional foundation branches joined in, and the campaign ran in every province. Then, in 2015, the GOHAVE1 campaign in British Columbia found an agreeable partner in Global Television. Female news anchors did spots to promote screening during an August campaign. A Global News story following up on that publicity burst boasted that the network had helped increase the number of screening mammograms by 30 percent from August a year earlier. The message and the news story were unequivocal about the necessity of getting screened. Dissenting voices were not included. The BC Cancer Agency teamed up with Global again in 2016 to run a similar campaign in October — and again reported a boost in mammogram bookings.

Here's the problem. The orange-versus-seed scenario hyperbolizes. In the real world, the average size of tumours women can feel is about two centimetres, slightly larger in diameter than a Canadian nickel. Most invasive cancers detected by mammograms are between one and one-and-a-half centimetres. Of course, mammograms may reveal smaller tumours, but it would just as surely be unusual for a woman not to feel something before it becomes the size of an orange. The Canadian Breast Cancer Foundation merged with the Canadian Cancer Society in 2017, but the GOHAVE1 video with phone number linked to provincial screening programs continued to exist on the merged website for several months in 2018.

Seeing clearly through the information blur from screening programs and fundraising organizations, compounded by competing guidelines from different medical organizations — the American Cancer Society versus the US Preventive Services Task Force, for example — is not easy. Being told vaguely that screening saves lives isn't helpful if you aren't also being told about the costs, about the harms you might endure as well as the benefits. The risks of dying of breast cancer, and the harms and benefits of screening, need to be quantified in a meaningful way. A bald statement that mammography screening reduces deaths from breast cancer by 25 percent makes it seem that the benefits are huge. But it represents a proportion and tells us nothing about the absolute numbers. Imagine a study that finds that eating an apple a day cuts your risk of toenail fungus by 50 percent. That's a relative reduction in risk. But if only two people out of a thousand ever get toenail fungus, the absolute risk is 0.2 percent. If eating an apple a day cuts that risk by 50 percent, the absolute risk is reduced to 0.1 percent. If you know only the relative difference in risk, 50 percent, you might stock up on apples. But if you know your absolute risk of toenail fungus is reduced by only 0.1 percent, you might decide it's perfectly fine to mix in some oranges with those apples.

With mammograms and breast cancer, unless you know the actual number of deaths reduced, it's impossible to know whether a 25 percent reduction is a little or a lot. Consider some numbers provided by the US Preventive Services Task Force when it updated its mammography screening recommendations in January 2016. Based on data from the randomized trials, the task force estimated the number of deaths prevented by screening ten thousand women regularly for ten years. In women aged forty to forty-nine, screening would prevent four deaths. Screening would prevent eight deaths in women aged fifty to fifty-nine, twenty-one deaths in women aged sixty to sixty-nine, and thirteen deaths in women aged seventy to seventy-four. In all, there would be forty-six fewer deaths among ten thousand women screened for ten years compared to ten thousand women not screened.

The task force observed another important finding from the randomized trials. When measuring the mortality benefit of an intervention, in this case repeated breast screening, it's useful to know not just how many women died of breast cancer but also how many women died of something else. If, for some reason, more or fewer women in the screened group than in controls died of another cause, that could provide more information about the benefits or harms of screening. Suppose more screened women died of another form of cancer. That would raise a whole other set of questions. If an intervention reduces death from one cause, it truly has benefit only when the total mortality from all causes also goes down. In the task force's analysis, screening had no impact on all-cause mortality.

The Canadian equivalent of the US Preventive Services Task Force is the Canadian Task Force on Preventive Health Care. It also strives to provide complete, clear information with absolute numbers, designed for physicians and the lay public and easily accessible on its website. The original version of the Canadian task force disbanded in 2005 due to a lack of funds, but the Canadian government revived it in 2010, instituting a panel of fourteen experts, who, like the members of the US task force, are all volunteers. Reincarnated, the new Canadian Task Force on Preventive Health Care made breast-screening guidelines its first priority.

The first chair of the re-established Canadian task force was Marcello Tonelli, a kidney specialist and a senior associate dean of medicine at the University of Calgary. From medical school at Western University and Dalhousie University, he went on to complete a master's degree in clinical epidemiology at Harvard in 2002. He's youthful and enthusiastic about evidence-based decision making and the importance of independent bodies setting guidelines in preventive medicine. Under his leadership, the task force decided to begin its work by revising the breast-screening guidelines, now ten years old and out of date, especially after the US task force revised its recommendations in 2009. Also, breast screening was a good example of where the analysis and decision tools the task force could provide would be useful. "There's been an evolution across the board with screening generally, from a simplistic 'Do this; it will save your life' message to a much more nuanced message that is more appropriate for most services," Tonelli explains. And if you're starting something new, he adds, you might as well start with something people will notice.

The task force wanted to put the true benefits and true harms of screening in perspective. Tonelli finds an analogy in parachutes. "There are some data you just don't need to have a discussion about. There may not be great studies about whether parachutes are helpful, but if we jump out of a plane, we don't need to talk about it. Put on your parachute, shut up, and jump out of the plane." Breast cancer screening is not like a parachute, he says, but people talk about it as if it is. "Generally speaking, benefits with screening are small. And generally speaking, the benefits of screening are overstated, and the harms are understated." Tonelli understands that people overstate the benefits because fundamentally they are optimistic, believing it makes sense to catch a disease early. But their simple message, "Ladies, get your mammogram," is inappropriate.

The Canadian task force released its new guidelines in November 2011,[1] recommending against routine mammography screening for women aged forty to forty-nine. This was a change. In 2001, the task force said the evidence wasn't strong enough either in favour of or against screening and recommended only that, beginning at age forty, women should be told about the benefits and risks and assisted in deciding when to begin screening. The task force also revised its long-standing recommendation that women aged fifty to sixty-nine be screened annually. It now recommended routine screening every two to three years but stated that the absolute benefits were small. "Women aged fifty to sixty-nine who do not place a high value on a small reduction in mortality and who are concerned about false-positive results, unnecessary diagnostic testing and potential overdiagnosis of breast cancer are likely to decline screening," the panel reported in the *Canadian Medical Association Journal*. It made the same recommendation for women aged seventy to seventy-four, with the same caveats. On its website, the task force provides some essential details, clearly outlining the absolute benefits and risks. The contrast between the detailed information offered by independent panels looking systematically at the evidence and the superficial information offered by many organizations vested in screening — cancer agencies, screening programs, and radiology groups — is striking. Not surprisingly, the Canadian task force guidelines met strong opposition.

---

1   As this book was going into print, the task force was revising the 2011 breast-screening guidelines, with an update due at an unspecified time in 2018. The update will reflect new research on the harms and benefits of screening, and research on how women weigh those harms and benefits when making screening choices.

The Canadian Breast Cancer Foundation leapt into the fray. The foundation was a natural ally in screening advocacy and awarded funds for screening research and imaging equipment. In 2009, it had hosted an event called "It's About Time! A Consensus Conference" to bring together breast cancer survivors, research scientists, health care providers, and government representatives to hear from twenty-one experts on early detection of breast cancer. The conference was Martin Yaffe's idea, and he headed its scientific advisory committee. Also on the advisory board was Roberta Jong, the director of breast imaging at Sunnybrook and a radiologist who, like Yaffe, once had a connection to the Canadian National Breast Screening Study and had become a foe. The other three advisory group members were Etta Pisano, director of the Biomedical Research Imaging Center at the University of North Carolina School of Medicine; Kathleen Pritchard, a clinical epidemiologist at Sunnybrook Research Institute and clinical director of the Ontario Clinical Oncology Group who was also a member of the board of directors of the Canadian Breast Cancer Foundation; and Robert Smith, director of cancer screening at the American Cancer Society. This was an advisory committee heavily weighted in favour of screening.

To call this a consensus conference was a misnomer as it wasn't about arriving at any kind of consensus among divergent views. It was designed more as a way to extol the virtues of screening and diagnostic technology. It was about doing early detection better, about new technologies, and, Yaffe wrote, about how women could get more information on "how they could best avoid being diagnosed with advanced breast cancer." In the end, the Canadian Breast Cancer Foundation made recommendations that included screening average-risk women annually from ages forty to fifty-five and every one or two years thereafter. Most screening programs in Canada did not actively recruit women in their forties, although some programs accepted them with physician referrals.

Not surprisingly, then, the Canadian Breast Cancer Foundation was ready to respond when the Canadian Task Force on Preventive Health Care unveiled recommendations to begin screening at age fifty. "We're really disappointed in these recommendations," its chief executive officer, Sandra Palmaro, told the *Globe and Mail*. "They're ultimately going to result in more women dying from breast cancer that don't need to be dying from breast cancer." The foundation's position was that all provinces should provide women ages forty to forty-nine with access to mammography screening programs. In a press release, it declared: "Strong scientific evidence and the public demand exists for screening Canadian women aged forty to forty-nine for breast cancer." The release quoted radiologist Paula Gordon: "Our own data from BC show twenty-five to thirty-nine per cent mortality reduction among screened women aged forty to forty-nine." How those numbers were calculated was not explained. The foundation objected that the task force relied on data from screening trials that were twenty-five to forty years old and had used outdated equipment. This was partly true. The trials were old, but the data the task force relied on were not. The trial investigators had continued to collect data on the women in their studies, tracing how many were eventually diagnosed with breast cancer and how many died, for many years after the screening phases of the trials ended.

In the media, reaction to the task force focused mainly on the recommendation not to screen women in their forties. The *National Post*, for example, featured a testimonial from a forty-five-year-old woman in Mississauga, Ontario, who declared she was the luckiest person in the world because a mammogram saved her life. But the real story might have been the task force's conclusion that although mammography screening reduces mortality, the absolute benefit for women of any age, the actual number of lives saved, is small. Most of the debate had centred on whether or not to screen younger women, as if screening women over fifty was indisputable. But in light of the evidence, asking at what age it is best to start screening might not have been the right question. It might have been better to ask whether screening should happen at all.

Peter Gøtzsche congratulated the Canadian task force for guidelines that "are more balanced and more in accordance with the evidence than any previous recommendations." In an editorial for the *Canadian*

Medical Association Journal, he wrote, "if screening had been a drug, it would have been withdrawn from the market," and asked, "Which country will be the first to stop mammography screening?" But, he argued, the task force hadn't looked at all the relevant research. It had concentrated on the randomized trials to assess the effect on mortality, but there were now important observational studies to consider. Observational studies differ from randomized trials because they simply observe what is happening in a population, as opposed to testing an intervention by assigning people randomly to either a group that gets the intervention or a control group. For example, you might follow a large group of thirty-year-olds and collect data on their socio-economic status and lifestyle habits, such as diet, exercise, alcohol, or smoking. You would also collect data on who develops heart disease or high blood pressure, gets any kind of cancer, succumbs to diabetes, and so on. Such a study might follow this group for decades, finally collecting mortality statistics to identify any correlation between behaviours, such as smoking, and cause of death. In the hierarchy of studies, observational research ranks lower than the gold standard randomized trial but can nevertheless provide useful information.

A unique situation in Denmark provided an excellent opportunity for observational research. As previously noted, screening was offered in the early 1990s in certain counties in Denmark for women aged fifty to sixty-nine, accounting for only 20 percent of women in that age group. The rest of Denmark did not institute screening for another seventeen years. As a consequence, women fell into either a screened group or an unscreened group by virtue of geography, resulting in a kind of natural experiment and a gold mine of data. Karsten Jørgensen, working with Gøtzsche and others at the Nordic Cochrane Centre, analyzed that data and found that mortality from breast cancer was similar in both groups, with a 1 percent reduction in mortality in the screened areas and a 2 percent reduction in mortality in the non-screened areas. Jørgensen reported the findings in the *BMJ* in 2010. Another study in the *BMJ*, in 2011, compared neighbouring nations with similar medical care where screening was introduced ten or fifteen years later in one than in the other. Researchers compared Northern Ireland to the Republic of Ireland, the Netherlands to Belgium, and Sweden to Norway. The fall in breast cancer mortality was about the same in each comparison.

Gøtzsche suggested that the observed mortality reduction had more to do with treatment than with screening. New therapies, such as tamoxifen, came along at about the same time that population screening became popular. Even before screening began, women were more aware of their breasts and were going to doctors earlier when they felt a lump. In Denmark, the average tumour at the time of detection decreased by nearly a centimetre between 1979 and 1989. Certainly, in Europe as well as North America, breast cancer mortality has decreased markedly since the mid-1980s. In Canada, the annual breast cancer mortality rate in 1986 was thirty-two per one hundred thousand women, and in 2015, it was down to less than eighteen in one hundred thousand women. What part screening could have played and what part better treatment is impossible to say with certainty, but the comparisons between areas with screening and areas without are persuasive. Even the screening advocates acknowledge that treatment has played a role in breast cancer outcome.

On its website, the Canadian Task Force on Preventive Health Care provides a discussion tool to help doctors discuss breast screening with patients. It's a good tool as long as doctors know about it. Karen Delaney-Laupacis was aware of the task force and its guidelines when she went to her family doctor not long after they were issued. She saw a resident at a family practice clinic in a Toronto hospital. He noticed that she had turned fifty and wanted her to get a mammogram. Delaney-Laupacis, a nurse who is interested in evidence-based medicine, also knew the guidelines suggested that doctors should discuss the benefits and risks with their patients. But this resident knew nothing about the task force and just said, "We like everyone to get a mammogram." Delaney-Laupacis didn't do it and has since chosen to attend another family clinic. The anecdote illustrates that it's not just patients who are susceptible to the pervasive early-detection messaging.

In fact, doctors in Ontario get the message reinforced directly by their government, through financial incentive. They make more money when their patients consent to screening. It doesn't happen anywhere else in Canada, but such incentive schemes also exist in the United States. In 1999, the Ontario Ministry of Health and Long-Term Care introduced an alternative to the traditional fee-for-service payments to family physicians. It set up a system where certain types of family practice clinics or health networks could enter into payment contracts with the ministry and would be eligible for pay-for-performance allocations. The Ontario pay-for-performance scheme, or P4P, is modelled after a system in Britain. Most family practitioners in the province receive bonuses when they involve a threshold number of patients in specific preventive care measures. Colonoscopies, cervical cancer screening, and mammograms are on the list of several measures that apply. If 75 percent or more of patients invited to breast screening answer the call, the bonus is $2,200. If fewer patients comply, the bonus decreases according to a sliding scale. It might not be a lot of money, but it sends a clear signal that screening is an important health measure. That it's a standard of care is further emphasized in the "MyPractice: Primary Care" reports doctors can choose to receive annually. The reports let doctors know how well they are doing with cancer screening and offer tips on how to improve.

Jennifer Young is a family physician in Collingwood, Ontario, and president-elect of the Ontario College of Family Physicians. She qualifies for the incentive bonuses. Speaking personally, in no way making any kind of statement on behalf of the college, she doesn't believe she should be pushing mammograms. In her practice, she prefers the more balanced approach the Canadian task force recommends, in which she has a discussion with patients about the limited benefit of breast screening and the potential for overdiagnosis and other harms. She generally has an interest in "less is more" medicine and concerns about overtesting and overmedicalizing in the current environment, where both patients and doctors believe more is better. She hates turning people into patients unnecessarily. Since 2011, Young has been conducting Practising Wisely workshops for members of the college. The workshops deal with the harms of too much medicine, with an emphasis on overprescribed drugs, polypharmacy (the concurrent use of multiple medications, a common problem in treatment of the elderly), overmonitoring of diabetes, and cancer screening. Of all the things discussed in a two-day workshop, she finds that doctors react the most to breast screening. "They're all, 'Oh my God, really?' They can't believe that the data for mammograms is almost as bad as for PSA tests. Of all the messages in the course, that's the biggest one for them." But then they'll ask, "What about the Ontario government incentivizing us to get women screened?"

Young would not tell a woman to skip screening. She'll introduce the subject, even when women don't yet have their invitation letter, but she has a discussion that aims for a shared decision process. She thinks about half of her patients still go for it, and that's their right: she just wants them to have the information. And, as she points out, she doesn't get paid for that. "Everything is pushing us to do mammograms," she says, "not to have a discussion."

The attempt to quell discussion is a consistent undercurrent throughout the mammography story. John Bailar felt resistance from his bosses at the NCI when he raised questions about the Breast Cancer Detection Demonstration Project. Daniel Kopans wrote to Barry Kramer's boss at the NCI and to the White House to complain that the journal Kramer edited was biased. Anthony Miller had to defend his research against an accusation of scientific misconduct. Michael Baum was met with stony silence when he questioned the way Britain was running its breast screening program. Donald Berry felt shunned at an academic conference. At a public event where Cornelia Baines tried to talk about the excess deaths among screened women early in the Canadian study, a radiologist jumped up to accuse her of being unethical and irrational. Peter Gøtzsche had a battle getting his Cochrane review published. US Preventive Services Task Force members have been accused of murdering women when their conclusions about breast screening didn't align with conventional wisdom.

Add the name Mette Kalager to the list of scientists screening advocates attempted to silence. Kalager was a surgeon who started out in a local county hospital in Norway and found herself drawn to breast cancer surgery. Then the hospital changed the way it handled breast cancer patients. Instead of a system of ad hoc assignments based on whoever was available, a senior surgeon was dedicated to all the breast cancer patients. The hospital adopted a multidisciplinary team approach to each patient, and she could see that this might improve outcomes. Observing the impact of a change in practice inspired an interest in research, and Kalager decided to get a PhD in medicine. She also wanted to return to Oslo, where she had earned her medical degree. She canvassed people she knew in the breast surgical community and suddenly received an offer to direct the Norwegian breast screening program, administered by the Cancer Registry of Norway. That was in 2004. She would steward the breast screening program at the same time she evaluated and conducted a research project on it. She was head of the program until 2006 and then became a researcher with the cancer registry.

Her first project was to assess whether the Norwegian program was fulfilling the expectation it would save lives. As in Denmark, circumstances in Norway resulted in an excellent source of observational data. Norway instituted screening gradually in 1996, expanding its program across the country over the next nine years. When Kalager compared death rates from breast cancer in counties where women were offered screening to those counties that didn't yet have it, she found a 10 percent reduction in mortality among women screened. But screening alone could account for only a third of that reduction. Mortality rates in unscreened women had also improved, possibly due to better care.

At first, Kalager couldn't believe what she saw. She and the more senior people she was working with, including the head of the cancer registry, were taken aback, despite indications elsewhere that mammography screening might not be as good as they thought. They went back and forth over the data. Co-workers at the registry were shocked too, and in a meeting to discuss the results, Kalager could feel that people were emotional and angry. They didn't want to hear what she had to say about her analysis; they wanted only to find problems with it. It felt like an inquisition.

Kalager's next project was to estimate the rate of overdiagnosis by comparing the number of invasive cancers detected in the screened areas in Norway to the number in unscreened areas. For the first number of years in a screening program, there will always be more cancers detected among screened women because of lead time. Mammograms detect cancers early, but after two to five years, the number of diagnosed cancers in the comparison group should even out if there is no overdiagnosis from screening. After accounting for lead time and other variables, Kalager was able to estimate that screening in Norway resulted in a rate of overdiagnosis ranging from 18 percent to 25 percent, meaning that up to one in four cancers diagnosed through screening might not have gone on to do any harm. She counted only invasive cancers; DCIS did not factor in the analysis. These results were in keeping with similar research in Denmark, where Karsten Jørgensen had reported in 2009 that, including DCIS, one in three cancers detected through screening were overdiagnosed. Kalager was planning to publish her results and was ready to submit her PhD thesis to the University of Oslo. The university organized a three-person committee that would read the material, provide a written evaluation, and then hear Kalager's defence. But the usual course of events did not happen. The committee asked her to take out everything she'd written about overdiagnosis.

Kalager was stunned. She protested that she should have the chance to have a discussion and defend her research. She hadn't been given the reasons why the committee thought her analysis was not correct. She suggested to her dean that one of the committee members had a conflict of interest because of her own pronouncements in favour of screening. Getting nowhere with her arguments, Kalager made the difficult decision to withdraw the overdiagnosis research. She felt, however, that she couldn't write the thesis summary without a section on benefits and harms. But when she submitted it, her work was once again rejected. She was now even more convinced that what was happening was all wrong. Unwilling to accept what she thought was a violation of academic freedom, she hired lawyers and engaged her union in her fight. Meanwhile, the *Annals of Internal Medicine* had agreed to publish

Jørgensen found the incidence of advanced cancer diagnoses to be the same in both. Incidences of DCIS and smaller, non-advanced cancers were substantially greater in the screened group. He estimated that overdiagnosis of those cancers occurred in one of every three cases, although there was a range depending on age, regional differences, and whether DCIS was counted in the analysis. Also, because it was an observational study and not a randomized trial, he couldn't be sure that the women in the screened areas were exactly comparable to the women in unscreened areas.

Measuring overdiagnosis is immensely complicated. With so many factors at play, there can never be one correct number, says Jørgensen. How often screening takes place, for instance, whether every year or every two or three, can produce different results. How well the screening is done and how well the mammograms are read are factors. In some screening programs, the false positive and call-back rates are higher than in others. Age at screening is important because overdiagnosis is more likely in women over seventy. In Denmark, a group of researchers known to be proponents of the country's screening program debates Jørgensen's findings. They've estimated that only 2.3 percent of breast cancers are overdiagnosed. Other researchers have used mathematical modelling to come up with rates of overdiagnosis. The tricky part about modelling is that you can obtain different results depending on which assumptions you choose to plug in. In general, the use of modelling has produced lower overdiagnosis estimates.

In the United States, where there aren't organized public screening programs, estimating overdiagnosis is especially difficult. Gilbert Welch, an epidemiologist and professor in the Department of Family and Community Medicine at the Dartmouth Institute in New Hampshire, has written countless articles on the problem of overdiagnosis across all of medicine, in a number of diseases. In 2012, he co-authored a study that estimated that 1.3 million American women had been overdiagnosed in three decades of mammography screening, and in one year, 2008, overdiagnosis accounted for 31 percent of breast cancers diagnosed. It needs to be highlighted that, due to limitations in the data, these are best guesses. For one thing, it wasn't possible to tell which breast cancers were detected through screening. However, the three decades offered a clear, big-picture view. If you detect cancers at an early stage, the number of advanced cancers you detect should go down. The teeter-totter should balance. But the incidence of advanced cancers remained the same.

Four years later, Welch led a study into the effectiveness of mammography screening versus breast cancer treatment in reducing mortality. The study concluded that systemic therapy was the predominant factor in improved survival, not screening. And again, US data showed that although screening has resulted in the detection of a higher number of small tumours, the incidence of metastatic cancer has not gone down. Contrary to arguments from screening advocates such as Paula Gordon or Daniel Kopans that overdiagnosis is greatly exaggerated, the data showed that it is substantial, of a magnitude larger than is generally recognized, although, again, estimates are imprecise because overdiagnosis cannot be directly measured.

The lack of clarity around overdiagnosis may be a reason screening programs offer so little information about it. In Canada, the Quebec screening program is alone in attempting to quantify it in a meaningful way. Most women who receive the brochures that come with screening invitations will be told only that "some" cancers will not go on to cause any harm — if they read that far into the brochure. The word *overdiagnosis* might not even appear. That's certainly the case in Ontario. But brochures are the work of bureaucrats and public relations consultants. In the real world of clinics, cold machines, and fear, generalities often do not apply. Derek Muradali, the Ontario breast screening program's chief radiologist, is forthcoming when he sits down in front of his computer screen to illustrate what he looks for on a mammogram. "You need to know what you're getting yourself into," he says. Some cancers can be missed. "Even if you find a little tiny breast cancer like this," he adds, pointing to a small blot of white on the screen, "that cancer may sit there for twenty years and may not cause the death of the woman, it may not affect her, she may die with it and never know about it. So some cancers that we find may never cause a woman's death. It's an overdiagnosis. We find too many of those." Even if overdiagnosis can't be precisely counted, it's a recognized problem.

Screening program leaflets also downplay the psychological cost of false positive results and biopsies that prove negative. Screening enthusiasts such as Paula Gordon feel that the harm of short-term anxiety is justifiable if lives are saved. But the anxiety might not be so short term. John Brodersen argues that it is too easily and cavalierly dismissed. Brodersen is a professor of public health at the University of Copenhagen and a general practitioner. While training, he observed a surgeon giving women the results of their breast biopsies. It didn't matter, he noticed, whether the surgeon told them they had breast cancer or they were healthy; they'd had a false positive result from the mammogram. "It was the same reaction, they all started crying, they all had a terrible time, but to those diagnosed with breast cancer, he said, you will have to talk to the nurse and she will give an appointment, so you will come next week and we will make a plan for your treatment. While to those having a false positive he just said bye bye." Brodersen wondered *what happens now* to these women? Who is taking care of *them*? The question affected him so intensely it became the subject of his doctoral thesis in 2006. Since then, he has undertaken several studies of the psychosocial consequences of false positive results and has found that women can suffer from anxiety that affects work, income, sexual function, sleep, relationships, and general health for up to three years after such a brush with breast cancer. In fact, the psychological impact is almost as severe as it is with women who have a confirmed diagnosis followed by treatment. As a result of screening, healthy, well-functioning women join the ranks of the "worried well." "My point is we change these women as people," Brodersen says. "We have even done a qualitative study, four to five years after screening mammography, and they still report that it has changed their life."

Exacerbating the information gap is the tendency for women to overestimate the risk of dying of breast cancer. The pink campaigns each October, breast screening programs, and radiology groups are good at exploiting women's fear of the disease. Breast cancer is a scourge that still kills about five thousand women each year in Canada; that cannot be denied. But that number has remained stable over the last few decades, even as the population has increased. To put it in perspective, consider that in 2012, 22,865 women died of heart disease, 7,543 of stroke, and 4,825 from accidental causes. And although it's most often said that the lifetime risk of having invasive breast cancer is one in nine, in reality, a Canadian woman who is fifty to fifty-five years old has a risk of one in four hundred, and a woman who is sixty-five to seventy has a risk of one in 285. The lifetime risk of dying from breast cancer is one in thirty. The same is true for women in the United States. To tell women that one in nine will have cancer paints a scary picture, but it's incomplete. It is true that breast cancer is a leading cause of death in younger women, and that's one of the reasons it conjures up so much fear and emotion. It is cruel and terrible when women die prematurely in their forties, fifties, or sixties. We would like it not to happen. It's why early detection offered so much promise.

When Anthony Miller and then Cornelia Baines began their journey into the breast screening world so many years ago, they thought, and hoped, mammography screening would save countless women from horrible death. Their research obliged them to let go of that belief, while the breast screening community turned its back on them and attacked their study relentlessly. Asked today whether women should get screened, Miller says he wouldn't recommend it; women should be aware of their breasts and see their doctors if they have concerns. Baines would just like women to know the truth about mammography's limitations. "I would be happy if women were able to make a totally, honestly, informed choice."

Depending on their own values and their level of cancer anxiety, women may wish to take their chances with the roulette of harm versus benefit. But Cornelia Baines would say they should be trusted with the ability to assess balanced information and make up their own minds.

Conclusion   IF NOT MAMMOGRAMS, WHAT?

The mantra of early detection became a creed a very long time ago. The debate over the "facts" is unlikely ever to be resolved because it's about belief, not science. Belief born sincerely out of a desire to save women from a horrible, premature death. Belief born from hope and perpetuated by vested interests. No medical practice is as controversial or political as breast screening.

After decades of debate since the 1960s HIP study, after the screening trials involving six hundred thousand women that took place in the 1980s, and after all the reviews from expert independent panels, it appears evident that if screening delivered anything beyond what improved treatments have accomplished over the last three decades, it is minimal. None of eight randomized trials in the United States, Canada, Sweden, and Scotland showed any statistically significant benefit of screening for women in their forties. Researchers in England conducted a ninth trial in the 1990s. Called the Age Trial, it recruited only women aged thirty-nine to forty-one and followed them for ten years. One hundred sixty thousand women were randomly assigned to annual screening or to a control group. The results showed no difference in mortality. In the Canadian National Breast Screening Study, women aged fifty to fifty-nine screened by mammography plus a physical breast exam had the same mortality outcome as women screened by physical exam alone. In the other trials, mammography reduced mortality in women aged fifty to sixty-nine by 15 to 30 percent at most. No matter how you look at it, a test that results in a good outcome 15, 20, or even 30 percent of the time is far from perfect and made all that more poor when you factor in the side effects. Moreover, although there might have been a reduction in deaths from breast cancer, the research tells us that all-cause mortality was not affected. That's the true test of efficacy. None of the breast screening trials was perfect, and the technology of the 1980s is not the technology of today. Still, if early detection truly worked, the data should support it unequivocally.

Will screening ever stop? It's highly unlikely, at least not any time soon. The infrastructure is too entrenched. And with any effort to stop screening, women would feel that something is being taken away from them. Witness the politics in the United States when the US Preventive Services Task Force did not recommend screening for women in their forties. The ensuing uproar resulted in the government legislating insurance companies to pay for it anyway. A good percentage of US women screened are in their eighties, some even when they are terminally ill from some other cause. Screening is an entitlement that will not easily be withdrawn. An ad in the New York subway, spotted in January 2018, says a great deal about what feeds that entitlement. A woman clutches the nipple of a bare breast, and underneath, on her rib cage, a strip that resembles an adhesive bandage reads, "I'm covered." The banner on the ad, in big, bold letters, reads, "Free preventive mammograms," as if a mammogram is a vaccine that will prevent a woman from contracting cancer. The ad's sponsor is Oscar, a health insurance company.

A recent flare-up in England illustrated anew how engrained the early detection mantra continues to be and how political it is. On Wednesday, May 2, 2018, UK Health Secretary Jeremy Hunt stood in the House of Commons to make an announcement. Due to a computer failure dating back to 2009, 450,000 women in England failed to receive their final invitation to screening when they were between the ages of sixty-eight and seventy-one. He said it was unclear whether any delay in diagnosis resulted in avoidable harm or death, but he was ordering an independent review to determine the clinical impact. It was estimated that between 135 and 270 may have had their life shortened because of the error, but Hunt clarified that the estimate was based on statistical modelling, and there was no clinical consensus on what benefits there were from screening in these older women. He said, however: "Tragically there are likely to be some people in this group who would have been alive today if the failure had not happened." The next day thousands of women clogged an information hotline set up to answer their questions. The immediate reflexive reaction was to shout "scandal" and "disaster." It took another day in the news cycle before calmer voices were heard reminding people that screening brought harms as well as benefits and that women shouldn't rush to get a catch-up mammogram.

Although screening as public policy is unlikely to come to a full stop, it is coming under increasing scrutiny. When the American Cancer Society altered its guidelines to recommend that women begin screening at forty-five, not forty, it was a signal change. In the United Kingdom, although there is strong government support for screening, the Marmot review, and public pressure, resulted in more balanced information leaflets. In Switzerland and in France, independent reviews of the evidence have resulted in calls for major rethinking.

The Swiss Medical Board came to a surprising conclusion in a report made public in 2014. The board is an independent health technology assessment initiative sponsored by the Conference of Health Ministers of the Swiss Cantons, the Swiss Medical Association, and the Swiss Academy of Medical Sciences. Asked to conduct a review of mammography screening, it recommended that no new programs be initiated and there be a time limit on existing programs. Only eleven of Switzerland's twenty-six cantons, or federal states, had established systematic screening program up to that point, two of them just in the previous year. In an April 2014 *New England Journal of Medicine* article, two of the board members explained the recommendations, with the caveat that they were speaking for themselves, not for all board members. They were struck by the fact that the randomized trials were old and wondered if the modest mortality benefit would still be found in a trial conducted today, in an era of more modern treatment. They were impressed by "how nonobvious it was that the benefits of mammography screening outweighed the harms" and disconcerted by a pronounced discrepancy between women's perceptions of the benefits and the benefits in reality. "It is easy to promote mammography screening if the majority of women believe that it prevents or reduces the risk of getting breast cancer and saves many lives through early detection of aggressive tumours," the authors wrote. "We would be in favour of mammography screening if these beliefs were valid. Unfortunately, they are not and we believe women should be told so." The Swiss Medical Board has the power only to make recommendations. Even so, the report infuriated screening advocates.

Peter Jüni was one of the members of the board and one of the authors of the *New England Journal of Medicine* article. A clinical epidemiologist, he has since moved to Toronto and is now the director of the Applied Health Research Centre at St. Michael's Hospital and a professor at the University of Toronto. The recommendation not to introduce new screening programs was radioactive, says Jüni. Not only did it create an angry flurry in the Swiss media, but it also generated strong reaction from US radiologists. As he observed the emotional outcry, he realized that much of it was coming from people who did not know, or did not want to believe, the data. But he was incredulous when an esteemed colleague reacted in that same unthinking way, and he decided to speak out. Jüni doesn't mind if women opt for screening if they've been made aware of all the evidence. What he objects to is women being told "fairy tales."

In France, the minister of health asked the French National Cancer Institute to conduct a review of breast screening through a public consultation process involving citizens, patients' organizations, charities, health professionals, government institutions, and screening experts. Such a wide public consultation was a bold alternative to the usual reviews conducted by experts. It took a year. A national screening program had been introduced in 2004 for women over fifty, but there were organizational problems, issues with access, and concerns about overdiagnosis and overtreatment. The cancer institute summarized the consultation results in October 2016, concluding that there was no scientific consensus about the benefits and risks of screening. Women were not getting information about the uncertainties, there was confusion between primary prevention and early diagnosis, and "outrageous pink October marketing" was misleading. It recommended no reimbursement for screening to women under fifty and suggested overhauling the program to offer women over fifty individualized screening based on their own risk factors. In April 2017, the health minister put forward a plan for reform to be implemented over the next several years. The new program would encourage women to make their own decisions with support from their doctors. Each woman over fifty would have a consultation where cancer screening options and risk reduction through lifestyle changes would be discussed. Invitations to screening would come with a booklet of complete information, with more resources offered online. Doctors would receive training to enable them to discuss the benefits, risks, and limitations of screening. The approach would make mammography personal.

If not mammography screening, what? Researchers such as Daniel Kopans and Martin Yaffe are hoping that 3-D mammography, also called DBT, which is commonly used in diagnostic workups of breast cancer, might prove to be a better tool for screening than the current mammography. It is increasingly used for screening in the United States, although there isn't yet enough evidence of its merits to convince the US Preventive Services Task Force or other expert panels. Research so far suggests that DBT is more sensitive than regular mammography, but the technique involves slightly higher radiation exposure. Since radiation, even from regular mammograms, is known to cause rare breast cancers, the imaging industry is working on refining DBT to address this concern.

Other researchers are strongly promoting MRI screening, but the panels are unconvinced about that, too, because of a high rate of false positives and the cost. Christiane Kuhl, a radiology professor at Bonn University, is testing a more efficient "abbreviated" MRI, involving far less time in the MRI machine and providing images that radiologists can read in a matter of seconds. Steven Narod, however, worries about an even higher rate of overdiagnosis should MRI become used in screening. He is among the many screening critics who argue that the quest for ever-earlier detection, as the answer to mammography's limitations, is misguided. Technology is not the problem, Narod insists. "Early detection is not helpful for breast cancer." Meanwhile, a few scientists are continuing to investigate possible markers for breast cancer, for instance, in blood. They are working on "liquid biopsies," tests to find tumour cells, or tumour DNA, circulating in blood, hoping in this way to detect a number of different cancers. This research is far from clinical application.

What about the clinical breast exam, which worked well in the Canadian trial? In terms of cancer detection, mammography did better than the clinical exam, but the clinical exam combined with mammography did better than mammography alone. In terms of mortality, there was no difference. However, clinical breast exams are not considered practical. In the Canadian study, the exam took from five to fifteen minutes depending on the breast density, the examiner's experience, and other factors — far too long for today's visit to the doctor's office. But more importantly, clinical exams require expertise and if poorly done can send many women for tests they don't need or miss things that need investigation. The nurses in the Canadian study were trained. The monthly breast self-exam, so urgently pressed upon women just a few years ago? Studies have shown that it doesn't have any effect on mortality. These days, women are advised to be "breast aware." Look for changes in the shape of the breast, for any wrinkling or dimpling, and watch for lumps. Obsession is not required.

There is much interest in individualized screening based on personal risk, and the study Laura Esserman is conducting in California, where genetics will help identify risk, will be closely watched. Research to solve the DCIS conundrum, sorting out which early cancers may or may not develop, like the study Shelley Hwang in North Carolina is doing, should yield important information. Two similar DCIS studies are under way in Europe. If we can somehow separate innocent DCIS, or innocent invasive cancer, from cancer we know will grow, we might be able to reduce the rates of overdiagnosis.

Not touched upon in this book is the question of how we prevent breast cancer from happening in the first place. Some suggest that is where the focus should be, or at least that there should be more emphasis in that direction. Screening costs a lot money: $8 billion annually in the United States, £100 million in England, €220 million each year in Germany, $20 million a year in British Columbia, and many more millions in Ontario. Advocacy groups such as Breast Cancer Action in California ask why more isn't spent on looking at the environmental causes of breast cancer.

The mammogram story is full of rancour and ugly debate in which good scientists have been shunned and bullied and women have been misled if not lied to. It's a lesson in how paradigms, once established, become inflexible, resistant to new insights and questions. At the same time, one positive and important result of the early detection doctrine, at least with regard to breast cancer, is how much it has done to raise awareness. Gone are the dark ages, not so long ago, when women were ashamed and kept breast cancer a secret, afraid of going to their doctors and thus delaying treatment. Awareness brings with it consumer pressure that demands better treatment and better research. But a paradigm that seemed to work in the 1980s and 1990s has been proven faulty and even harmful. An approach that treats everyone as if they are exactly the same, as if we all have the same values, risks, and fears, is not supportable. Mass population screening was a well-meant strategy, born in another era. No well-informed woman who understands the nuances in the knowledge we have today and who wants to say no to screening mammograms should feel guilty. It is a reasonable choice.

References

Cornelia Baines and Anthony Miller granted extensive interviews and provided access to their files and private papers. Other interviewees include Halya Kuchmij, Derek Muradali, Richard Strax, John C. Bailar, Myron Moskowitz, Charles Wright, Peter Scholefield, Ed Sickles, David Beatty, Daniel Kopans, Martin Yaffe, Sharon Batt, Suzanne Fletcher, Cindy Pearson, Barnett Kramer, Richard Klausner, Donald Berry, Kay Dickersin, Connie Rufenbarger, Fran Visco, Penny Gerrie, Peter Gøtzsche, Ned Calonge, Diana Petitti, John Keen, Michael Linver, Leonard Berlin, Paula Gordon, Terry Minuk, Therese Taylor, Karla Kerlikowske, Jan Vick Harris, Desiree Basila, Shelley Hwang, Steven Narod, Hazel Thornton, Michael Baum, Julietta Patnick, Karsten Jørgensen, John Brodersen, Iona Heath, Fiona Godlee, Marcello Tonelli, Karen Delaney-Laupacis, Jennifer Young, Mette Kalager, and Peter Jüni. Imogen Evans answered questions via email. Thanks also to many people who do not appear in the book but who were also interviewed and provided information and insight. They include Teresa To and Claus Wall from the Canadian National Breast Screening Study; John Wasson, Daniel Sullivan, and Laurie Fajardo, members of the 1997 Consensus Development Conference; Virginia Moyer, former chair of the US Preventive Services Task Force; James Dickinson and Neil Bell, former members of the Canadian Task Force on Preventive Health Care; surgeon Richard Margolese; radiologist Jill Wruble; family physician Michelle Albert-Burke; medical oncologist Ellen Warner; health consumer advocate Maryann Napoli; breast cancer survivor Susanne Reber; Rita Weil, daughter of Philip Strax; radiologist Linda Warren; Gregory Doyle, chair of the Canadian Breast Screening Network; Anne Kearney, health policy researcher; and Suzie Joanisse, former administrator, Ontario Breast Screening Program.

Introduction

Maureen Roberts's essay, "Breast Screening: Time for a Rethink?" was published in the *BMJ*, vol. 299, no. 6708, on November 4, 1989.

The Regina Hospital in Hastings, Minnesota, has been hosting mingle and mammogram parties since the fall of 2010. Notices for the parties appear in the *Cornerstone*, the hospital foundation's newsletter, at https://www.allinahealth.org/uploadedFiles/Content/Business_units/Regina_Hospital/160328RG-Cornerstone-newsletter.pdf.

Sheryl Crow's relationship with Hologic is described in *Health News Review*, published on July 19, 2016, and available at https://www.healthnewsreview.org/2016/07/sheryl-crow-hawks-3-d-mammograms-with-fear-and-false-hope/.

The updated results of the Canadian National Breast Screening Study can be found at Miller et al., "Twenty Five Year Follow-up for Breast Cancer Incidence and Mortality of the Canadian National Breast Screening Study: Randomised Screening Trial," published in the *BMJ*, vol. 348, February 12, 2014. The *BMJ* paper was the subject of many international media stories. For the *New York Times* front-page article, see "Vast Study Cast Doubts on Value of Mammograms," by Gina Kolata, the *New York Times*, February 12, 2014.

Chapter 1

Under Sydenham Skies, by Cornelia Johanna Baines (Markham, ON: Fitzhenry and Whiteside, 2001).

David Sackett, the head of the program at McMaster University where Cornelia Baines studied, died on May 13, 2015, at age eighty. Toronto's *Globe and Mail* published an extensive obituary. Sackett completed medical school at the University of Illinois in 1959 and in the 1960s worked for the US Public Health Service until he was wooed to McMaster in 1967. He founded the university's clinical epidemiology department and remained there until he went to the University of Oxford in England and established the International Centre for Evidence-Based Medicine. His work influenced many of the people who appear in this book.

Video of President Nixon signing the National Cancer Act is available on YouTube, courtesy of the National Cancer Institute (https://www.youtube.com/watch?v=E2dzEDnGqHY).

The Canadian Ad Hoc Committee on Mammography presented its report in the *Journal of the Canadian Association of Radiologists*, vol. 25, no. 1, March 1974.

For the first results from the Health Insurance Plan of Greater New York study, see Strax, Venet, and Shapiro, "Value of Mammography in Reduction of Mortality from Breast Cancer in Mass Screening," in *American Journal of Roentgenology*, vol. 117, no. 3, March 1973.

The problems with Irwin Bross are detailed in "Mammography Study A Mistake," *Canadian Family Physician*, vol. 26, January 1980. In the *American Journal of Public Health*, vol. 69, no. 2, February 1979, an editorial note accompanying an article by Bross et al. said Bross "stands virtually alone in his data and the interpretations he places on them." Because of the media attention Bross had been getting, the journal departed from its usual policy to print only peer-reviewed material, which Bross would not allow. The *Globe and Mail* published the letter from Bross on November 28, 1979. "100,000 Guinea Pigs Sought for Cancer Fight," by Margaret Munro, was published in the *Ottawa Citizen* on November 29, 1979. Bross continued his campaign against the Canadian National Breast Screening Study in a letter to *CMAJ*, vol. 123, July 19, 1980.

Baines and Miller reached out to physicians in "The Canadian National Breast Screening Study: Why It Deserves Support," published in *Canadian Family Physician*, vol. 28, March 1982. Miller's editorial in the same issue is titled "The National Breast Screening Study: An Opportunity for Family Physicians." Cornelia Baines documented efforts to improve recruitment into the breast screening study in "Impediment to Recruitment in the Canadian National Breast Screening Study: Response and Resolution" in *Controlled Clinical Trials*, vol. 5, June 1984.

The *Sunday Times* article "Breast Scans Boost Risk of Cancer Deaths," by John Cassidy and Tim Rayment, was on the newspaper's front page on June 2, 1991. The *Lancet* editorial that followed appeared in vol. 337, June 29, 1991.

For the review of the Canadian study's mammograms, see Baines et al., "Canadian National Breast Screening Study: Assessment of Technical Quality by External Review," in *American Journal of Roentgenology*, vol. 155, October 1990. The commentary by Daniel Kopans, in the same issue, is titled "The Canadian Screening Program: A Different Perspective."

The quoted newspaper headlines are from the *Toronto Star*. "Despite Breast Cancer Study, Save Your Life and Get Tested" headlined a column by Michele Landsberg, published on November 19, 1992. "Breast X-rays Still Urged, Mammograms Useful Despite Study Results, MD," headlined a report by Nicolaas van Rijn, published on November 15, 1992. "Doctors Defend Breast X-rays," by Lisa Priest, appeared on November 17, 1992.

Chapter 2

The early history of mammography is well documented in *A History of Cancer Control in the United States, 1946-1971* (Washington, DC: National Cancer Institute, Division of Cancer Control and Rehabilitation, 1979), in two volumes prepared by the History of Cancer Control Project, UCLA School of Public Health, with Lester Breslow as principal investigator. Book One, Chapter 5, is devoted to the role of mammograms in detecting breast cancer. Also see "Highlights from the History of Mammography," by R.H. Gold, L.W. Bassett, and B.E. Widoff, in *RadioGraphics*, vol. 10, no. 6, November 1990. Richard Gold's summary, "The Evolution of Mammography," can be found in the transcript for the NIH/NCI Consensus Development Meeting on Breast Cancer Screening in 1977, available from the HathiTrust digital library (https://hdl.handle.net/2027/purl.32754081211041), on page 61.

For the study looking at the reproducibility of Egan's work, see Clark et al., "Reproducibility of the Technic of Mammography (Egan) for Cancer of the Breast," in *American Journal of Surgery*, vol. 109, February 1965.

Details about Philip Strax were provided by interviews with members of the family, who also shared the bound transcript of a commissioned interview done by Ellen Robinson Epstein of the Center of Oral History, November 20, 1990, in Washington, DC, when Strax was eighty-one. The bound transcript includes the recommendation letter his teacher wrote to assist him in obtaining scholarships. The Florida newspaper *Sun Sentinel* published a feature about Strax on August 14, 1988, when he won the Kettering Prize for cancer research. Strax's book, *Early Detection: Breast Cancer Is Curable* (New York: Harper and Row, 1974), contains photographs of early mammography machines.

For early results from the HIP study, see Shapiro et al., "Evaluation of Periodic Breast Cancer Screening with Mammography," *JAMA*, vol. 195, no. 9, February 28, 1966. For later results, see Shapiro et al., "Periodic Breast Cancer Screening in Reducing Mortality From Breast Cancer," *JAMA*, vol. 215, no. 11, March 15, 1971.

Information about Arthur Holleb is from *The Breast Cancer Wars: Fear, Hope, and the Pursuit of a Cure in Twentieth-Century America*, by Barron H. Lerner (Oxford: Oxford University Press, 2001); from Lerner's article, "'To See Today With the Eyes of Tomorrow': A History of Screening Mammography," in *Canadian Bulletin of Medical History*, vol. 20, no. 2, 2003; from *The Big Squeeze: A Social and Political History of the Controversial Mammogram*, by Handel Reynolds (Ithaca, New York: ILR Press, 2012); from *Unnatural History: Breast Cancer and American Society*, by Robert. A. Aronowitz (New York: Cambridge University Press, 2007); and from "Presumptive Risks Should Not Nullify Benefits of Mammography, Holleb Says," an article in *The Cancer Letter*, vol. 4, no. 29, July 21, 1978. The American Cancer Society press release, "Toward Better Control of Breast Cancer," issued by Holleb on October 4, 1971, is cited by Lerner.

The early history of the Pap test is described in *A History of Cancer Control in the United States, 1946-1971*, and its importance to the American Cancer Society is described in an interview with pathologist Leopold Koss. He said it was a society without a cause until someone had the genius idea to propagate the cervical smear. The Pap test's importance to the American Cancer Society is also described in *Crusade: The Official History of the American Cancer Society*, by Walter Ross (New York: Arbor House, 1987), and in other books, including *Unnatural History: Breast Cancer and American Society*, by Aronowitz. The Kodak and Picker x-ray ads are cited by Lerner.

Nathaniel Berlin's interview with the NCI oral history project took place on June 30, 1997.

Barron Lerner wrote about the "Betty Ford blip" in a blog titled "Not So Simple: The Breast Cancer Stories of Betty Ford and Happy Rockefeller" for the *Huffington Post*, published September 26, 2014 (https://www. huffingtonpost.com/barron-h-lerner/not-so-simple-the-breast-_b_5733402.html).

Chapter 3

In addition to the author's interviews with John Bailar, an invaluable source was "A Conversation with John C. Bailar III," by Susan Ellenberg in *Statistical Science*, vol. 12, no. 2, May 1997.

A source for much of this chapter is the full transcript of the NIH/NCI Consensus Development Meeting on Breast Cancer Screening, September 1977, cited earlier, available from the HathiTrust digital library. A document prepared in March 1977 in advance of the meeting, "Final Reports of National Cancer Institute Ad Hoc Working Groups on Mammography Screening for Breast Cancer and a Summary Report of Their Joint Findings and Recommendations," was later published in the *Journal of the National Cancer Institute*, vol. 59, no. 2, August 1977. The consensus development meeting was the first of dozens of such meetings on a variety of health measures, and its experimental nature is described in Donald Fredrickson's foreword to the published transcript. The NIH ended its consensus development program in 2013.

Rose Kushner told her own story in *Breast Cancer: A Personal History & an Investigative Report* (New York: Harcourt Brace Jovanovich, 1975). Obituaries in the *New York Times* and *Washington Post* and the article "No Shrinking Violet: Rose Kushner and the Rise of American Breast Cancer Activism," by Barron Lerner, in the *Western Journal of Medicine*, vol. 174, no. 5, 2001, provided additional information.

For a summary of the interim screening guidelines issued to the demonstration project screening centres, as well as a chronology of events leading to the NIH consensus development meeting, see Diane Fink's presentation in the above-cited transcript, pages 7-19. She was then director of the Division of Cancer Control and Rehabilitation at the NCI. A detailed chronology was also provided in a background statement prepared for the consensus development meeting.

John C. Bailar's "Mammography: A Contrary View" was published in the *Annals of Internal Medicine*, vol. 84, no. 1, January 1976. He expanded his arguments in "Screening for Early Breast Cancer: Pros and Cons," *Cancer*, vol. 39, June supplement, 1977.

The controversies leading up to the 1977 consensus conference, including the Sidney Wolfe revelations and Jack Anderson's column, are documented in Lerner's *The Breast Cancer Wars*. Some details are also documented in "Breast Cancer: Second Thoughts about Routine Mammography," by Barbara Culliton in *Science*, vol. 193, August

13, 1976. Daniel S. Greenberg chronicled the developing controversy in "X-Ray Mammography — Background to a Decision," in the *New England Journal of Medicine*, vol. 295, no. 13, September 23, 1976.

Jane Brody's article, "Mammography Test for Cancer in Women Under 50 Defended," was published in the *New York Times* on July 20, 1976.

For Arthur Holleb's definition of high-risk women, see his editorial, "Restoring Confidence in Mammography," in *CA: A Cancer Journal for Clinicians*, vol. 26, no. 6, November/December 1976.

Many thinks to Barbara Faye Harkins, archivist in the Office of NIH History, for digging up photos of the Masur Auditorium from around the time the consensus meeting took place.

John Bailar's articles about the "War on Cancer" in the *New England Journal of Medicine* are "Progress against Cancer?" co-authored with Elaine M. Smith and published in vol. 314 on May 8, 1986, and "Cancer Undefeated," co-authored with Heather L. Gornik and published in vol. 336 on May 29, 1997.

Chapter 4

Much of the information in this chapter comes from documents and correspondence provided by Cornelia Baines and Anthony Miller, including Miller's doctoral thesis and his own unpublished biographical work. Baines's files contain minutes from the study's policy advisory group meetings and from annual meetings of the study's surgeons and radiologists. (Before discovering these files, the author attempted for several months to access the policy advisory group minutes now housed in the Canadian Cancer Society archives. Even though the Canadian National Breast Screening Study was publicly funded and the documents are three decades old, the author was told these historic documents could not be made public.)

The GE television ad appeared in a CBC documentary in 1991; other ads mentioned were collected by Charles Wright.

The American Cancer Society provides a history of its cancer screening guidelines on its website (https://www.cancer.org/health-care-professionals/american-cancer-society-prevention-early-detection-guidelines/overview/chronological-history-of-acs-recommendations.html).

Charles Wright's article in *Surgery*, "Breast Cancer Screening: A Different Look at the Evidence," is in vol. 100, no. 4, October 1, 1986. The report from the Swedish Two-County trial by Tabár et al., "Reduction in Mortality from Breast Cancer after Mass Screening with Mammography," is in the *Lancet*, vol. 325, no. 8433, April 13, 1985.

Nancy Reagan's memoir, *My Turn* (New York: Random House, 1989), contains a chapter on her breast cancer, quoting her diary entries. Additional details are from the *New York Times*, October 18, 1987, and March 5, 1988, and from *The Big Squeeze: A Social and Political History of the Controversial Mammogram*, by Handel Reynolds.

Cornelia Baines's observations about the differences between the Swedish Two-County trial and the Canadian trial are documented in "Rational and Irrational Issues in Breast Cancer Screening," *Cancers*, vol. 3, no. 1, March 2011.

A Canadian Press story describing what László Tabár said at the breast cancer symposium in Banff, Alberta, titled "Breast Debate Deadly," appeared in the *Winnipeg Sun* on April 30, 1986.

Details regarding the mammography equipment used in the Canadian breast screening study and the types of views taken are in "Canadian National Breast Screening Study: Assessment of Technical Quality by External Review," by Baines et al., *American Journal of Roentgenology*, vol. 155, no. 4, October 1990. The review, conducted in 1988, was unprecedented. No other mammography trial was subject to such intense scrutiny. Daniel Kopans's dissenting view, in the same issue, was published as a commentary titled "The Canadian Screening Program: A Different Perspective." The journal published the rebuttal to Kopans by Miller, Baines, and Sickles in its letters section, vol. 155, no. 5, November 1990.

Chapter 5

A video of Daniel Kopans at the Radiological Society of North America meeting on December 3, 2014, appears on YouTube (https://www.youtube.com/watch?v=LzLA9ovXGYc&t=182s). The origin of "Aunt Minnie" is explained at https://www.auntminnie.com.

Journalist Gary Taubes wrote about the mammography debate in "The Breast Screening Brawl," *Science*, vol. 275, no. 5303, February 21, 1997. In an accompanying article in the same issue, he profiled Kopans and his extreme views in "How One Radiologist Turns Up the Heat."

The paper Kopans denounces in the AuntMinnie.com interview is A. Bleyer, H.G. Welch, "Effect of Three Decades of Screening

Mammography on Breast-Cancer Incidence," *New England Journal of Medicine*, vol. 367, no. 21, November 22, 2012.

"Women Who Have Breast Scanning Are More Likely to Die of Cancer" was published in London's *Sunday Times* on June 2, 1991. Julietta Patnick, National Coordinator, England's National Breast Screening Programme, Sheffield, wrote her letter to the editor denouncing the Canadian study as flawed on June 9, 1991. The story was also picked up by Victoria Macdonald in the *Sunday Telegraph* on June 9, 1991. A debate in the *Lancet* over the *Sunday Times* article began with an editorial published in vol. 337, June 29, 1991. Miller's reply was in vol. 338, July 13, 1991, and Kopans's reply was in vol. 338, August 17, 1991. Debate in the *Journal of the National Cancer Institute* began with an article in vol. 84, no. 11, June 3, 1992, "Author of Canadian Breast Study Retracts Warnings." Responses from Miller, Kopans, and others were published in vol. 84, no. 17, September 2, 1992.

The National Medical Roundtable on Mammography and the variations in guidelines from different organizations are discussed by Handel Reynolds in *The Big Squeeze*. Details on American Cancer Society guidelines and on the roundtable are also provided by Gerald Dodd in "American Cancer Society Guidelines on Screening for Breast Cancer: An Overview," *CA: A Cancer Journal for Clinicians*, vol. 42, no. 3, May/June 1992.

Gina Kolata's story, "Doubts Increase on Need for Early Mammogram," *New York Times*, March 1988, was in response to Eddy et al., "The Value of Mammography Screening in Women Under Age 50 Years, *JAMA*, vol. 259, no. 10, March 11, 1998. The *Washington Post* article, "New Study Expands Evidence on Benefits of Mammograms," September 21, 1988, reported on a study by Chu et al., "Analysis of Breast Cancer Mortality and Stage Distribution by Age for the Health Insurance Plan Clinical Trial," *Journal of the National Cancer Institute*, vol. 80, no. 14, September 21, 1988. "Mammogram Recommendation Draws Fire," published in the *Washington Post* on July 4, 1989, is a response to the roundtable consensus.

The observation that fewer than half of American women over fifty were getting mammograms is based on the results of the NCI Breast Cancer Screening Consortium and National Health Interview Survey Studies, reported in *JAMA*, vol. 264, no. 1, July 4, 1990, in an article titled "Screening Mammography: A Missed Clinical Opportunity?" Data from 1987 showed that only 25 to 41 percent of American women had had a mammogram in the previous year. The NCI's goal was to have 80 percent of women over fifty going for annual mammograms by 2000.

Barbara Bush's advocacy of mammography was reported by Lois Romano in "Barbara Bush, Prescribing Mammograms," *Washington Post*, September 21, 1989.

Cited Canadian media reports following the *Sunday Times* story are "Screening of Breasts Called Futile," by Rebecca Wood, *Vancouver Sun*, June 18, 1991; "Debate Rages Over Study on Breast Cancer," by Robin Harvey, *Toronto Star*, August 1991; and "Unpublished Breast-Cancer Study Sparks Furor," by Nicholas Regush, *Montreal Gazette*, September 21, 1991.

The workshop on early detection of breast cancer was reported in "Reducing Deaths from Breast Cancer in Canada," *CMAJ*, vol. 141, no. 3, August 1, 1989.

Canadian participation in breast screening, 1991, is detailed in a 1996 Health Canada report, "Organized Breast Screening Programs in Canada." Table 4, page 12, shows the rate for each year from 1988 to 1996. The report is available at http://publications.gc.ca/collections/collection_2011/sc-hc/H1-9-13-1996-eng.pdf.

Chapter 6

The Canadian National Breast Screening Study was published in the *CMAJ*, vol. 147, no. 10, November 15, 1992, in two parts: "Canadian National Breast Screening Study: 1. Breast Cancer Detection and Death Rates Among Women Aged 40 to 49 Years," and "Canadian National Breast Screening Study: 2. Breast Cancer Detection and Death Rates Among Women Aged 50 to 59 Years." In the conclusion of part two, Miller et al. explain that the results could change with a longer follow-up. Antoni Basinski's editorial appeared in the same issue of the *CMAJ*.

Martin Yaffe was misquoted in the news section of the *Journal of the National Cancer Institute*, vol. 84, no. 24, December 16, 1992. The journal printed a correction in vol. 85, no. 2, January 1993.

Reaction to the Canadian National Breast Screening Study from Ontario's chief medical officer Richard Schabas and Danielle J. Perrault, director of the Ontario Breast Screening Program, was issued by the Ontario Ministry of Health through Canada Newswire on December 16, 1992 ("Breast Cancer Screening — Making Sense Out of Confusion"). Brian

Goldman's opinion, responding to the flurry of comments in the media, appeared in *CMAJ*, vol. 148, no. 3, February 1, 1993. Responses from Warren and Burhenne, in the form of letters to the editor, were published in vol. 148, no. 6, March 15, 1993, along with a rebuttal from the study authors. In the media, the *Montreal Gazette* reported on the Association des radiologistes du Québec press conference on November 19, 1992, in a story titled "Mammography Study Flawed"; the Ontario Medical Association's comments were recorded in "Doctors Insist X-ray Breast Tests Still Needed," by Marilyn Dunlop in the *Toronto Star* on November 19, 1992; and comments from the head of the British Columbia breast screening program, Patricia Rebbeck, were published in *The Province* in "Cancer Study Puts Women at Risk: Critic," by Ann Rees, on November 15, 1992. Howard Seiden's analysis, "How Critics See Breast Cancer Study. Is This a War of Science or Simply Dirty Politics?," appeared in the *Toronto Star* on December 10, 1992, and in the *Hamilton Spectator* on December 26, 1992. There were many other media stories not mentioned in this chapter.

On December 15, 1992, Canadian Minister of Health Lucien Bouchard announced that the federal government would spend twenty-five million dollars over the next five years to fight breast cancer, most of it to fund research, but 2.3 million dollars would be devoted to provincial breast screening. This announcement came with the promise of an expert panel to review screening policy.

Sample US headlines are from newspapers dated either November 13 or November 14, 1992.

A contact of Cornelia Baines faxed to her on November 23, 1992, the memorandum sent to members of the American College of Radiology from its director of communications, written by Feig and Kopans and dated November 20, 1992. In May of that year, a US journalist sent Anthony Miller a memorandum, highly critical of the Canadian study but also erroneous, that Miller has been told was prepared in conjunction with a radiology conference in Boston.

The Fletchers' *Annals of Internal Medicine* article, "The Breast Is Close to the Heart," is in vol. 117, no. 11, December 1, 1992.

The paper Martin Yaffe and colleagues authored in *Radiology*, vol. 189, no. 3, December 1993, is titled "A Critical Appraisal of the Canadian National Breast Screening Study." Robert Tarone's paper, "The Excess of Patients with Advanced Breast Cancer in Young Women Screened with

Mammography in the Canadian National Breast Screening Study," is in *Cancer*, vol. 75, no. 4, February 15, 1995.

Bailar and MacMahon's review, "Randomization in the Canadian National Breast Screening Study: A Review for Evidence of Subversion," is in *CMAJ*, vol. 156, no. 2, January 15, 1997.

Kopans's paper in *Breast Cancer Research and Treatment*, "The Canadian National Breast Screening Studies Are Compromised and Their Results Are Unreliable. They Should Not Factor into Decisions About Breast Cancer Screening," is in vol. 165, no. 1, August 2017.

Chapter 7

Many of the details in this chapter concerning the NIH and the NCI are chronicled in "Four Decades of Mammography Wars," *The Cancer Letter*, April 24, 2015 (https://cancerletter.com/articles/20150424_3).

Sharon Batt is the author of *Patient No More* (Charlottetown, PEI: Gynergy Books, 1994).

Suzanne Fletcher et al.'s "Report of the International Workshop on Screening for Breast Cancer" appeared in *Journal of the National Cancer Institute*, vol. 85, no. 20, October 20, 1993.

The first report from the US Preventive Services Task Force was titled *Guide to Clinical Preventive Services: An Assessment of the Effectiveness of 169 Interventions* (Baltimore: Williams & Wilkins, 1989).

Reaction from Kopans to the results of the 1993 International Workshop on Screening for Breast Cancer was recorded in the *New York Times* article by Gina Kolata, February 26, 1993, and a CBC News story that aired on February 25, 1993.

Suzanne Fletcher reflected on reaction to the 1993 workshop in "Breast Cancer Screening: A 35-Year Perspective," published in *Epidemiologic Reviews*, vol. 33, 2011.

The American Cancer Society print ad appeared in *Mother Jones*, January 1990. The *Psycho* ad was featured in a CBC *Marketplace* documentary in 1991.

The chronology of the NCI's attempts to revise its guidelines and the quoted excerpts from those guidelines are in "Four Decades of Mammography Wars," *The Cancer Letter*, April 24, 2015.

The average cost of a mammogram was reported by Gina Kolata in the *New York Times*, quoting Larry Kessler, chief of applied research at NCI, on December 27, 1993.

Kopans's comment to *Science* was quoted in Gary Taubes, *Breast Screening Brawl* and *How One Radiologist Turns Up the Heat*, vol. 275, no. 5303, February 21, 1997.

Suzanne Fletcher summed up her observations about the 1997 consensus development conference in "Whither Scientific Deliberation in Health Policy Recommendations? — Alice in the Wonderland of Breast-Cancer Screening," *New England Journal of Medicine*, vol. 336, no. 16, May 1997.

The consensus development conference conclusions were reported in "Special Article, National Institutes of Health Consensus Development Conference Statement: Breast Cancer Screening for Women Ages 40-49, January 21-23, 1997," *Journal of the National Cancer Institute*, vol. 89, no. 14, July 16, 1997. Readers who wish to see abstracts from the conference speakers and other related articles in addition to the final conference statement may consult *JNCI Monographs*, vol. 1997, no. 22.

The fact that Leon Gordis was furious about what happened at the 1997 consensus conference was reported to the author by Kay Dickersin in an interview.

The Klausner quotation ("I was shocked") was reported by Gina Kolata in the *New York Times*, January 24, 1997. His statement at the press conference is from a transcript of his answers to reporters.

Klausner appeared before the Senate Appropriations Committee Subcommittee on Labor, Health and Human Services, Education, and Related Agencies on February 5, 1997.

Visco's statement to the Congressional hearings on mammography screening was addressed to Senator Specter.

Other sources for this chapter include the following:

Kay Dickersin, "Breast Screening in Women Aged 40–49 Years: What Next?," the *Lancet*, vol. 353, June 5, 1999.

Daniel Kopans, "The Breast Cancer Screening Controversy and the National Institutes of Health Consensus Development Conference on Breast Cancer Screening for Women Ages 40-49," *Radiology*, vol. 210, no. 1, 1999.

Bernadine Healy, "Editorial: Screening Mammography for Women in Their Forties: The Panel of Babel," *Journal of Women's Health*, vol. 6, no. 1, November 1, 1997.

"NCAB to Consider Mammography in Forties," Cancernetwork.com, March 1, 1997 (http://www.cancernetwork.com/articles/ncab-consider-mammography-forties).

Steven Woolf and Robert Lawrence, "Preserving Scientific Debate and Patient Choice: Lessons from the Consensus Panel on Mammography Screening," *JAMA*, vol. 278, no. 23, December 17, 1997.

N.J. Nelson, "The Mammography Consensus Jury Speaks Out," *Journal of the National Cancer Institute*, vol. 89, no. 5, March 5, 1997.

P. Eastman, "NCI Adopts New Mammography Screening Guidelines for Women," *Journal of the National Cancer Institute*, vol. 89, no. 8, April 16, 1997.

Chapter 8

Although public screening programs do not recommend screening women over seventy-four due to a lack of evidence supporting it, some medical organizations, such as the American College of Radiology, the Canadian Association of Radiologists, and the American Cancer Society, recommend that women seventy-five and older continue screening if they are in good health and are expected to live another ten years.

There is evidence that a first-degree (mother, sister) family history increases the risk of advanced breast cancer, even in older women, but the risk is small. See Dejana Braithwaite et al., "Family History and Breast Cancer Risk Among Older Women in the Breast Cancer Surveillance Consortium Cohort," *JAMA Internal Medicine*, vol. 178, no. 4, 2018.

By far the largest risk factor is age, and according to Engmann et al. in "Population-Attributable Risk Proportion of Clinical Risk Factors for Breast Cancer," in *JAMA Oncology*, published online February 2, 2017, data from a registry of women screened by mammography show that breast density in both pre-and post-menopausal women represents four to six times greater population-attributable risk of breast cancer than family history, and among post-menopausal women, obesity represents a population-attributable risk about four times greater than family history.

Gøtzsche describes the National Breast Cancer Coalition event in his book, *Mammography Screening: Truth, Lies and Controversy* (London: Radcliffe, 2012). Fran Visco also describes the standing ovation he received in a foreword to the book. The controversial *Lancet* article,

"Is Screening for Breast Cancer with Mammography Justifiable?," is in vol. 355, no. 9198, January 8, 2000.

For more about Archie Cochrane, see Georgios Dimitrakakis et al., "Archibald Cochrane (1909–1988): The Father of Evidence-Based Medicine," *Interactive Cardiovascular and Thoracic Surgery*, vol. 18, no. 1, January 1, 2014.

For more about Iain Chalmers, see Geoff Watts, "Iain Chalmers: Maverick Master of Medical Evidence," the *Lancet*, vol. 368, no. 9554, December 23, 2006.

The description of Peter Gøtzsche as a committed and meticulous scientist appears in Iona Heath's foreword to *Mammography Screening: Truth, Lies and Controversy*. A profile of Gøtzsche by Donald G. McNeil Jr. appears in "Confronting Cancer: Scientist At Work — Peter Gotzsche," *New York Times*, April 9, 2002. Gøtzsche's interview with John McDougall, dated April 1, 2015, is available at https://www.youtube.com/watch?v=paCAc9p_GsQ.

Swedish researchers G. Sjönell and L. Ståhle created an uproar with their paper "Mammographic Screening Does Not Significantly Reduce Breast Cancer Mortality in Swedish Daily Practice," *Läkartidningen*, vol. 96, no. 8, 1999.

Gøtzsche chronicles his research into mammography screening and the difficulties of getting his conclusions accepted in the above-cited book. He cites the newspaper articles about the Danish National Board of Health's reluctance to make public his report as A. Libak, "New Doubts About Breast Cancer Screening," and "The Danish National Board of Health Shelves Report," published May 20 and May 23, 1999, respectively, in *Berlingske Tidende*.

P. Gøtzsche and O. Olsen published their initial analysis in "Is Screening for Breast Cancer with Mammography Justifiable?," the *Lancet*, vol. 355, no. 9198, January 8, 2000. Letters to the editor responding to the article, including László Tabár's letter, co-authored with Stephen Duffy, appeared in vol. 355, February 26, 2000. The Cochrane breast cancer group editors responded in vol. 356, October 7, 2000. The Malmö study was discussed in Ingvar Andersson et al., "Mammographic Screening and Mortality from Breast Cancer: The Malmö Mammographic Screening Trial," the *BMJ*, vol. 297, October 15, 1988.

For the unapproved Nordic Cochrane review, see O. Olsen and P. Gøtzsche, "Cochrane Review on Screening for Breast Cancer with Mammography," and editor Richard Horton's commentary, "Screening Mammography— An Overview Revisited," in the *Lancet*, vol. 358, no. 9290, October 20, 2001. Replies to the editor's commentary, including a reply from the Cochrane Breast Cancer Group, are in vol. 359, no. 9304, February 2, 2002.

The 2006 Nordic Cochrane review, "Screening for Breast Cancer with Mammography," version 2, is available online at http://cochranelibrary-wiley.com/doi/10.1002/14651858.CD001877.pub2/full. The final review, version 5, published online in 2013, is at http://cochranelibrary-wiley.com/doi/10.1002/14651858.CD001877.pub5/full. All versions are also available at http://nordic.cochrane.org/research/cochrane-reviews.

The fact that lifetime risk of breast cancer death is 3 percent was obtained from *Canadian Cancer Statistics, 2017*, Government of Canada and Canadian Cancer Society and from *Cancer Facts and Statistics, 2018*, American Cancer Society.

Gina Kolata first wrote about Gøtzsche's controversial review in "Study Sets Off Debate Over Mammograms' Value," *New York Times*, December 9, 2001. The *New York Times* editorial, "The Latest Mammography Debate," followed on December 10, 2001.

The PDQ statement on screening resulted from a meeting on January 23, 2002, reported by Gina Kolata, "Expert Panel Cites Doubts on Mammogram's Worth," *New York Times*, January 24, 2002. The *New York Times* editorial, "Uncertainty Over Mammograms," was published on January 27, 2002. The PDQ board's opinion of Gøtzsche's analysis was reported by Faith McLellan in a news item in the *Lancet*, "Independent US Panel Fans Debate on Mammography," vol. 359, no. 9304, February 2. 2002.

Tommy Thompson's announcement in a press release from Health and Human Services, February 21, 2002, prompted another editorial from the *New York Times*, "The Latest Mammogram Report," February 27, 2002.

The National Breast Cancer Coalition published "The Mammography Screening Controversy: Questions and Answers," on April 16, 2002, on its website. The author received a copy from the coalition's archives. For a more up-to-date position statement still available on the coalition's website, see "Mammography for Breast Cancer Screening: Harm/Benefit Analysis Updated July 2011" at http://www.breastcancerdeadline2020.org/breast-cancer-information/

breast-cancer-information-and-positions/mammography-for-breast-cancer.pdf.

International Agency for Research on Cancer press release no. 139, March 19, 2002, "Mammography Screening Can Reduce Deaths from Breast Cancer," is available at https://www.iarc.fr/en/media-centre/pr/2002/pr139.html.

Cornelia Baines wrote about the Global Summit on Mammographic Screening in "Breast Practices," the *Medical Post*, June 25, 2002. The claims made by Tabár and Kopans at the summit are based on the following: Tabár et al., "Beyond Randomized Controlled Trials: Organized Mammographic Screening Substantially Reduces Breast Carcinoma Mortality," *Cancer*, vol. 91, no. 9, May 1, 2001, and J.S. Michaelson, E. Halpern, and D.B. Kopans, "Breast Cancer: Computer Simulation Method for Estimating Optimal Intervals for Screening," *Radiology*, vol. 212, no. 2, August 1999.

The antagonism Berry faced at the global summit is documented in correspondence with Cornelia Baines, the email from Peter Dean to Berry, March 21, 2002, and an interview with the author.

The editorial by Peter Boyle, "Global Summit on Mammographic Screening," was published in the *Annals of Oncology*, vol. 14, no. 8, August 2003.

The US Preventive Services Task Force recommendations on mammography screening were published in the *Annals of Internal Medicine*, vol. 151, no. 10, November 17, 2009.

Kathleen Sebelius's response to the US Preventive Services Task Force recommendations was reported by Kate Phillips in "Sebelius on Mammograms: Don't Change What You're Doing," *New York Times*, November 18, 2009.

Diana Petitti and Ned Calonge testifying and answering questions before the US House Energy and Commerce Subcommittee on Health can be seen at https://www.c-span.org/video/?290390-1/breast-cancer-screening-recommendations.

Chapter 9

For the updated Canadian research, see Miller et al., "Twenty Five Year Follow-up for Breast Cancer Incidence and Mortality of the Canadian National Breast Screening Study: Randomised Screening Trial," the *BMJ*, vol. 348, February 11, 2014. In an interview, Martin Yaffe criticized

Miller, arguing that treating the two parts of the study as one was a huge faux pas.

For the revised estimate of overdiagnosis in the National Breast Screening Study, see Baines, To, and Miller, "Revised Estimates of Overdiagnosis from the Canadian National Breast Screening Study," *Preventive Medicine*, vol. 90, 2016, June 2016.

Gina Kolata reported on the updated Canadian research in "Vast Study Casts Doubts on Value of Mammograms." Paula Gordon expressed her reaction in "Opinion: Shoddy Canadian Research Is Putting Women's Lives at Risk," *Vancouver Sun*, February 13, 2014.

The *BMJ* Rapid Responses to Miller et al. record an active debate through to the beginning of May 2014. They include comments from Daniel Kopans, February 12; László Tabár, February 18 and 20 and March 17; John Keen, February 17, and Miriam Pryke, March 14. Miller and/or Baines responded February 17, 19, 20, and 22 and March 10, 11, and 19. Per-Henrik Zahl reacted on February 12 to Tabár not declaring competing interests, citing C. Riva et al., "Effect of Population-Based Screening on Breast Cancer Mortality," the *Lancet*, vol. 379, 2012.

Michael Linver's response to Kolata's article in the *New York Times* appears at https://nyti.ms/2Lk6Pt4 and is one of 645 online comments.

Leonard Berlin and co-author Ferris Hall discussed the "mammography muddle" in "More Mammography Muddle: Emotions, Politics, Science, Costs, and Polarization," *Radiology*, vol. 255, no. 2, May 2010.

For the Coldman study, see Andrew Coldman et al., "Pan-Canadian Study of Mammography Screening and Mortality from Breast Cancer," *Journal of the National Cancer Institute*, vol. 106, no. 11, October 1, 2014. A response from Steven Narod, Vasily Giannakeas, and Miller appeared in the *Journal of the National Cancer Institute*, vol. 107, no. 5 (published online April 8, 2015).

The US Preventive Services Task Force draft recommendations on screening for breast cancer were released April 20, 2015. Final recommendations were published in the *Annals of Internal Medicine*, vol. 164, no. 4, February 16, 2016 (published online January 12, 2016), and are available at https://www.uspreventiveservicestaskforce.org/ Page/Document/UpdateSummaryFinal/breast-cancer-screening1. Kopans's reaction to the task force draft recommendations was posted on *AuntMinnie.com* April 21, 2015 (https://www.auntminnie.com/index. aspx?sec=sup&sub=wom&pag=dis&ItemID=110771).

The American Cancer Society's reaction to the task force's 2009 recommendations was reported by Gina Kolata in "Panel Urges Mammograms at 50, not 40," *New York Times*, November 16, 2009. The American Cancer Society's revised breast screening guidelines were published in *JAMA*, vol. 314, no. 15, October 20, 2015.

A list of media reaction to the American Cancer Society's revised guidelines was compiled by the Society of Breast Imaging at sbi-online.org (https://www.sbi-online.org/RESOURCES/ScreeningMammography/TabId/111/ArtMID/1322/ArticleID/75/American-Cancer-Society-Revises-Its-Mammogram-Guidelines.aspx). Robert Smith was quoted in *AuntMinnie.com*, October 20, 2015; the American College of Radiology's reaction appears in the same article, at https://www.auntminnie.com/index.aspx?sec=sup&sub=wom&pag=dis&ItemID=112175.

Cornelia Baines's description of her cancer appears in "Rethinking Breast Screening — Again," the *BMJ*, vol. 331, October 27, 2005.

Chapter 10

Breastcancer.org provides a good description of DCIS at http://www.breastcancer.org/symptoms/types/dcis. A comprehensive evaluation of the incidence, diagnosis, and treatment of DCIS is contained in "NIH State-of-the-Science Conference Statement on Diagnosis and Management of Ductal Carcinoma In Situ (DCIS)," *NIH Consensus and State-of-the-Science Statements*, vol. 26, no. 2, September 22-24, 2009. More recent evaluations include Mathias Worni et al., "Trends in Treatment Patterns and Outcomes for Ductal Carcinoma in Situ," *Journal of the National Cancer Institute*, vol. 107, no. 12, published online September 30, 2015; Tristen S. Park, Shelley Hwang, "Current Trends in the Management of Ductal Carcinoma In Situ," *Oncology Journal*, vol. 30, no. 9, September 15, 2016; and "Is the 'C' in DCIS Really Cancer?" a Breast Cancer Action webinar with Shelley Hwang, published February 15, 2017 (https://www.youtube.com/watch?v=yxewtb7RNfw). Statistics on DCIS survival come from the Ontario Breast Screening Program.

Mislabelling DCIS is discussed in Barbara K. Dunn, Sudhir Srivastava, and Barnett S. Kramer, "The Word 'Cancer': How Language Can Corrupt Thought," the *BMJ*, vol. 347, September 10, 2013.

"Milk Duct Tumours Not Really Cancer," by Lauran Neergaard of the Associated Press, appeared in the *Toronto Star,* September 25, 2009, a story about the NIH state-of-the-science statement on DCIS.

An abstract of Karla Kerlikowske's presentation to the NIH state-of-the-science panel on DCIS can be found at https://consensus.nih.gov/2009/dcisabstracts.htm#kerlikowske.

The National Heart, Lung, and Blood Institute of the NIH issued a clinical alert announcing the halt of the HRT trial on July 9, 2002 (https://www.nlm.nih.gov/databases/alerts/estrogen_progestin.html).

IDLE, a new nomenclature for indolent cancers, is discussed in the following: Laura Esserman, Yiwey Shieh, Ian Thompson, "Rethinking Screening for Breast Cancer," *JAMA,* vol. 302, no. 15, October 21, 2009; Laura Esserman, Ian Thompson, "Solving the Overdiagnosis Dilemma," *Journal of the National Cancer Institute,* vol. 102, no. 9, May 5, 2010; L.J. Esserman, I.M. Thompson Jr., B. Reid, "Overdiagnosis and Overtreatment in Cancer: An Opportunity for Improvement," *JAMA,* vol. 310, no. 8, August 28, 2013; and L.J. Esserman et al., "Addressing Overdiagnosis and Overtreatment in Cancer: A Prescription for Change," *Lancet Oncology,* vol. 15, no. 6, May 2014.

Jan Vick Harris's experience with DCIS is documented in "Ductal Carcinoma In Situ Stage 0 Breast Cancer: When Less May Be Better," *JAMA Internal Medicine,* vol. 176, no. 7, 2016 (published online May 31, 2016, and posted on the South Carolina Voices for Patient Safety Facebook page, January 22, 2017).

Details on the COMET trial are available at https://clinicaltrials.gov/ct2/show/NCT02926911.

An example of Esserman's research on molecular technology is provided here: Esserman et al., "Use of Molecular Tools to Identify Patients with Indolent Breast Cancers With Ultralow Risk Over 2 Decades," *JAMA Oncology,* vol. 3, no. 11, November 1, 2017. The WISDOM study is described in Esserman, "The WISDOM Study: Breaking the Deadlock in the Breast Cancer Screening Debate," *npj Breast Cancer,* published online September 13, 2017 (https://www.nature.com/articles/s41523-017-0035-5).

Criticisms of tailored screening and/or using SNPs appeared in the following: Stephen A. Feig, "Personalized Screening for Breast Cancer: A Wolf in Sheep's Clothing?" *American Journal of Roentgenology,* vol. 205, no. 6, December 2015; Steven A. Narod, "Breast Cancer Prevention in the Era of Precision Medicine," *Journal of the National Cancer Institute*, vol. 107, no. 5, May 1, 2015; and Daniel B. Kopans, "Breast Cancer Screening: Where Have We Been and Where Are We Going? A Personal Perspective Based on History, Data and Experience," *Clinical Imaging*, vol. 50, December 27, 2017.

The risk of breast cancer based on clinical data is reported in Engmann et al., "Population-Attributable Risk Proportion of Clinical Risk Factors for Breast Cancer," *JAMA Oncology*, vol. 3, no. 9, September 1, 2017. The estimate that 30 percent of women have a very low risk of breast cancer is in Kerlikowske et al., "Identifying Women With Dense Breasts at High Risk for Interval Cancer: A Cohort Study," *Annals of Internal Medicine*, vol. 162, no. 10, May 19, 2015 (see Table 1). The Breast Cancer Surveillance Consortium Risk Calculator can be found at http://tools. bcsc-scc.org/BC5yearRisk.

For Narod's research into DCIS, see Steven Narod et al., "Breast Cancer Mortality After a Diagnosis of Ductal Carcinoma In Situ," *JAMA Oncology*, vol. 1, no. 7, published online August 20, 2015. Similar findings from Shelley Hwang's team were reported in M. Worni et al., "Trends in Treatment Patterns and Outcomes for Ductal Carcinoma in Situ." Narod and team followed up their *JAMA Oncology* paper in a commentary, "Wherein the Authors Attempt to Minimize the Confusion Generated by Their Study," *Current Oncology*, vol. 24, no. 4, August 2017.

Narod explores the idea that breast cancer can disappear in "Disappearing Breast Cancers," *Current Oncology*, vol. 19, no. 2, April 2012. In this paper, he references P.H. Zahl et al., "Natural History of Breast Cancers Detected in the Swedish Mammography Screening Programme: A Cohort Study," *Lancet Oncology*, vol. 12, 2011.

Narod and Sopik presented their hypotheses in "Is Invasion a Necessary Step for Metastases in Breast Cancer?" published in *Breast Cancer Research and Treatment*, vol. 169, no. 1, May 2018. Readers may also like to see a critical response from Alan B. Hollingsworth and Narod's rebuttal letter, published in the June issue of the journal.

Chapter 11

Statistics on breast cancer deaths in the United Kingdom from the Forrest report appear in "Breast Cancer Screening: Report to the Health Ministers of England, Wales, Scotland and Northern Ireland,"

November 1986. On July 5, 1985, the *Guardian* reported that recommending a public screening service was a foregone conclusion when Patrick Forrest was asked to prepare the report. The government's announcement that it would establish a screening program was reported in the *Guardian* on February 25, 1987.

Hazel Thornton's article in the *Lancet*, "Breast Cancer Trials: A Patient's Viewpoint," is in vol. 339, no. 8784, January 4, 1992.

Testing Treatments was first published by The British Library in 2006. A revised edition was published by Pinter and Martin Ltd., London, in 2011.

Michael Baum's foreword to "After Screening: A Report on Diagnostic Services for Breast Cancer in the Greater London Area," by Sue Kerrison and Naomi Pfeffer, published by the Greater London Association of Community Health Councils, was quoted in the *Guardian* on April 20, 1990.

The article by C.J. Wright and C.B. Mueller, "Screening Mammography and Public Health Policy: The Need for Perspective," was published in the *Lancet*, vol. 346, no. 8966, July 1, 1995. Michael Baum responded in a letter to the editor, "Screening for Breast Cancer, Time to Think and Stop?," vol. 346, August 12, 1995.

Michael Baum described what happened at an emergency meeting of the national advisory committee to the screening program in an interview and had written about it in a letter to the *BMJ*, vol. 332, March 23, 2006, titled "Ramifications of Screening for Breast Cancer: Consent for Screening."

The UK screening program's participation statistics were reported in J. Chamberlain et al., "National Health Service Breast Screening Programme Results for 1991-2," *BMJ Clinical Research*, vol. 307, no. 6900, 1993.

Hazel Thornton questioned the value of screening and what women were being told in a presentation to the Fourth International Cambridge Conference on Breast Cancer Screening, April 4-6, 1995.

Jørgensen's research on website content is in Jørgensen and Gøtzsche, "Presentation on Websites of Possible Benefits and Harms from Screening for Breast Cancer: Cross Sectional Study," the *BMJ*, vol. 328, January 17, 2004. In that paper, the authors cited a Swedish report by L. Nyström et al., "Breast Cancer Screening with Mammography: Overview of Swedish Randomised Trials," the *Lancet*, vol. 341, no. 8851, 1993. Jørgensen and Gøtzsche's analysis of the content in invitations to publicly funded screening mammography appeared in the *BMJ*, vol. 332, no. 7540, March 2, 2006.

The Nordic Cochrane Centre published its critique of the UK breast screening leaflet in Gøtzsche et al., "Breast Screening: The Facts— or Maybe Not," the *BMJ*, vol. 338, January 28, 2009. Signatories to the letter to the editor of the *Times*, "Breast Cancer Screening Peril: Negative Consequences of the Breast Screening Programme," published February 19, 2009, included experts from the United States, Australia, and Canada as well as the United Kingdom. England's national cancer director's announcement of a formal review of screening invitations was reported by Zosia Chustecka in *Medscape News*, https://www.medscape.com/viewarticle/588786, February 26, 2009.

Iona Heath's article, "It Is Not Wrong to Say No," appeared in the *BMJ*, vol. 338, June 23, 2009.

Klim McPherson's article, "Screening for Breast Cancer—Balancing the Debate," appeared in the *BMJ*, vol. 340, June 24, 2010.

Julietta Patnick's defence of the December 2010 leaflet was quoted by Susan Mayor in "Critics Attack New NHS Breast Screening Leaflet for Failing to Address Harms," the *BMJ*, vol. 240, December 16, 2010. Her story also quoted Michael Baum, Peter Gøtzsche, and Valerie Beral. Beral told Mayor that the figures used in the leaflet came from a 2006 review, now archived at http://webarchive.nationalarchives.gov.uk/20150506043443/http://www.cancerscreening.nhs.uk/breastscreen/publications/nhsbsp61.pdf.

Susan Bewley's letter to Mike Richards, "The NHS Breast Screening Programme Needs Independent Review," and Mike Richards's response, "An Independent Review Is Under Way," are in the *BMJ*, vol. 343, October 25, 2011.

The Marmot report, "The Benefits and Harms of Breast Cancer Screening: An Independent Review," appeared in the *Lancet*, vol. 380, no. 9855, November 17, 2012 (online October 30, 2012). Michael Baum expressed his reaction to the report in "Harms from Breast Cancer Screening Outweigh Benefits If Death Caused by Treatment Is Included," the *BMJ*, vol. 346, January 23, 2013, and "The Marmot Report: Accepting the Poisoned Chalice," *British Journal of Cancer*, vol. 108, published online June 6, 2013. Peter Gøtzsche expressed his concern in a letter to the *Lancet*, vol. 381, March 9, 2013. Stephen Duffy also responded in a letter in the same issue.

The current National Health Service (England) breast screening leaflet is available at https://www.gov.uk/government/publications/breast-screening-helping-women-decide.

Fiona Godlee stated that she declined breast screening invitations when she gave the Elizabeth Blackwell Public Lecture at the University of Bristol on October 10, 2016, with the title: "Too Much Medicine: Why We Need to Push Back the Tide of Medical Excess."

Chapter 12

Samples of letters inviting women to screening in Ontario and the breast screening pamphlet are on Cancer Care Ontario's website (https://www.cancercareontario.ca/en). An example of a screening program's commitment to increase screening rates is also on that website (https://www.cancercareontario.ca/en/cancer-care-ontario/programs/screening-programs/ontario-breast-obsp), where it says, "To increase screening rates, we are working with the Ministry of Health and Long-Term Care and other partners to: more aggressively promote screening; use information technology and other supports to help primary care providers with screening; increase efforts to reach under-screened populations including new Canadians, people living in poverty, people without a family physician, First Nations, Métis, Inuit and other Aboriginal people. We aim to increase the proportion of Ontario women who have breast cancer screening, especially those from more vulnerable populations, by supporting local and regional innovative approaches to screening."

Information from the Quebec breast screening program, including its breast screening pamphlet, is available on the Government of Quebec website (http://sante.gouv.qc.ca/en/chroniques/avantages-inconvenients-et-limites-du-depistage-par-mammographie; http://publications.msss.gouv.qc.ca/msss/fichiers/2016/16-243-03A.pdf).

Although the Canadian Breast Cancer Foundation merged with the Canadian Cancer Society in 2017, the GOHAVE1 promotional video was accessible until the spring of 2018. The Global News story about the campaign is at globalnews.ca/tag/gohave1, and information about the partnership with Global and the results is available in annual Screening Mammography Program reports on the BC Cancer Agency's website (http://www.bccancer.bc.ca/screening/Documents/

SMP_Report-AnnualReport2016.pdf; www.bccancer.bc.ca/screening/
Documents/SMPAnnualReport2017_WEB.pdf).

The US Preventive Services Task Force analysis of breast cancer
mortality and all-cause mortality was reported in Heidi Nelson et
al., "Effectiveness of Breast Cancer Screening: Systematic Review
and Meta-analysis to Update the 2009 U.S. Preventive Services Task
Force Recommendation," *Annals of Internal Medicine*, vol. 164, no. 4,
published online January 12, 2016.

The Canadian Task Force on Preventive Health Care published "Recommendations on Screening for Breast Cancer in Average-Risk Women
Aged 40–74 Years," in the *CMAJ*, vol. 183, no. 17, November 22,
2011. The editorial by Peter Gøtzsche, "Time to Stop Mammography
Screening?," is in the same issue.

The Canadian Breast Cancer Foundation published "Earlier Detection
and Diagnosis of Breast Cancer: A Report from It's About Time! A
Consensus Conference" in October 2010. The report is available online
at https://www.cbcf.org/ontario/AboutBreastHealth/Documents/
CBCF+-+IAT+Report+Final[1].pdf.

The reaction to the Canadian Task Force on Preventive Health Care 2011
guidelines was reported in Carly Weeks, "New Breast Cancer Screening
Guidelines Inflame Debate, Add to Confusion," *Globe and Mail*,
November 21, 2011, and Tom Blackwell, "Mammograms at 40: I feel I
Was the Luckiest Person in the World," *National Post*, November 26,
2011. The Canadian Breast Cancer Foundation issued its press release
on November 21, 2011.

For the research comparing screened with unscreened women in
Denmark, see Jørgensen et al., "Breast Cancer Mortality in Organised
Mammography Screening in Denmark: A Comparative Study," the
BMJ, vol. 340, March 24, 2010. For comparisons in other countries,
see Philippe Autier et al., "Breast Cancer Mortality in Neighbouring
European Countries with Different Levels of Screening but Similar
Access to Treatment: Trend Analysis of WHO Mortality Database,"
the *BMJ*, vol. 343, July 28, 2011.

Gøtzsche's argument that treatments have more to do with reducing breast
cancer mortality than screening is in the above-cited *CMAJ* editorial.
Also see K.J. Jørgensen, J.D. Keen, P.C. Gøtzsche, "Is Mammographic
Screening Justifiable Considering Its Substantial Overdiagnosis Rate

and Minor Effect on Mortality?," *Radiology*, vol. 260, no. 3, September 2011.

Canadian breast cancer mortality statistics are reported annually in *Canadian Cancer Statistics*, published by the Government of Canada and the Canadian Cancer Society.

The Canadian Task Force on Preventive Health Care tools for discussion of breast cancer screening can be found at https://canadiantaskforce.ca/tools-resources/breast-cancer-2.

Regarding incentive payments to Ontario doctors, see T. Kiran et al., "Effect of Payment Incentives on Cancer Screening in Ontario Primary Care," *Annals of Family Medicine*, vol. 12, no. 4, July 2014, and J. Li et al., "Physician Response to Pay-for-Performance: Evidence from a Natural Experiment," *Health Economics*, vol. 23, no. 8, August 2014. A sample "MyPractice" report is provided by Health Quality Ontario (http://www.hqontario.ca/Quality-Improvement/Guides-Tools-and-Practice-Reports/Primary-Care).

For Mette Kalager's research on breast screening in Norway, see M. Kalager et al., "Effect of Screening Mammography in Breast-Cancer Mortality in Norway," *New England Journal of Medicine*, vol. 363, no. 13, September 23, 2010. Also see "Overdiagnosis of Invasive Breast Cancer due to Mammography Screening: Results from the Norwegian Screening Program," *Annals of Internal Medicine*, vol. 156, no. 7, April 3, 2012.

Jørgensen's analyses of overdiagnosis can be found in "Overdiagnosis in Organised Mammography Screening in Denmark. A Comparative Study," *BMC Women's Health*, vol. 9, no. 36, December 22, 2009, and in "Breast Cancer Screening in Denmark, A Cohort Study of Tumor Size and Overdiagnosis," *Annals of Internal Medicine*, vol. 166, no. 5, January 10, 2017. A lower rate of overdiagnosis is reported by A.B. Beau et al., "Benefit-to-Harm Ratio of the Danish Breast Cancer Screening Programme," *International Journal of Cancer*, vol. 141, no. 3, August 1, 2017.

For Gilbert Welch's work on overdiagnosis, see A. Bleyer, H.G. Welch, "Effect of Three Decades of Screening Mammography on Breast-Cancer Incidence," *New England Journal of Medicine*, vol. 367, no. 21, November 22, 2012, and H.G. Welch et al., "Breast-Cancer Tumor Size, Overdiagnosis, and Mammography Screening Effectiveness," *New England Journal of Medicine*, vol. 375, no. 15, October 13, 2016.

For John Brodersen's research on the psychological harms of screening, see "Long-Term Psychosocial Consequences of False-Positive Screening Mammography," *Annals of Family Medicine*, vol. 11, no. 2, March/April 2013.

Mortality rate statistics are quoted from Statistics Canada.

Conclusion

The Age Trial was reported in Sue Moss et al., "Effect on Mammographic Screening from Age 40 Years on Breast Cancer Mortality at 10 Years' Follow-up: A Randomised Controlled Trial," the *Lancet*, vol. 368, no. 9552, December 9, 2006. A mortality benefit in the women screened was not statistically significant.

Analysis of all-cause mortality in the screening trials was referenced in Chapter 12: Heidi Nelson et al.

The New York subway ad "I'm covered" was the subject of a report by *Health News Review*, January 25, 2018 (https://www.healthnewsreview. org/2018/01/patients-doctors-journalists-criticize-free-preventive-mammograms-campaign).

The breast screening error in England was the subject of numerous media reports, including "The Computer Glitch That Led to 450,000 Cancelled Breast Screenings," by Sarah Boseley, in the *Guardian*, May 2, 2018, and "Breast Cancer Screening Helpline Inundated with Calls," also by Boseley, in the *Guardian*, May 4, 2018; "Breast Screening: What Went Wrong?," BBC News, May 2, 2018; "Health Chiefs Blame Each Other Over Cancer Test Failure," by Chris Smyth, in the *Times*, May 3, 2018; and "Women Are Urged to Avoid Catch-up Breast Screening," also by Smyth in the *Times*, May 5, 2018.

The Swiss Medical Board report was discussed in N. Biller-Andorno and P. Jüni, "Abolishing Mammography Screening Programs? A View from the Swiss Medical Board," *New England Journal of Medicine*, vol. 370, no. 21, May 22, 2014. A summary of the board's recommendations can be found at http://www.medical-board.ch/fileadmin/docs/public/mb/fachberichte/2013-12-15_bericht_mammographie_final_kurzfassung_e.pdf.

The breast screening program debate in France was reported in G. Moutel et al., "Women's Participation in Breast Cancer Screening in France — An Ethical Approach," *BMC Medical Ethics*, vol. 15, no. 64, 2014; "Plan d'action pour la rénovation du dépistage oganisé du cancer du sein,"

Institut National du Cancer, April 2017 (http://solidarites-sante.
gouv.fr/IMG/pdf/plan-actions-renov-cancer-sein-2.pdf); A. Barratt,
K.J. Jørgensen, and P. Autier, "Reform of the National Screening
Mammography Program in France," *JAMA Internal Medicine*, vol. 178,
no. 2, 2018; and Roxanne Nelson, "Make Screening Mammography
Personal, Say the French," published November 3, 2017, and available
at https://www.medscape.com/viewarticle/888005.

The cost of screening in the United States was estimated by Cristina
O'Donoghue et al., "Aggregate Cost of Mammography Screening in
the United States: Comparison of Current Practice and Advocated
Guidelines," *Annals of Internal Medicine*, vol. 160, no. 3, February
4, 2014. In England, the annual cost of the National Health Service
breast screening program is cited as £96 million by Fiona Godlee in
"Breast Screening Controversy Continues," the *BMJ*, vol. 346, January
24, 2013. The cost in Germany was reported by Astrid Eich-Krohm in
"The Mammography Screening Debate in Germany: Yes or No?" *Breast
Cancer Consortium*, August 15, 2014 (http://breastcancerconsortium.
net/mammography-screening-debate-germany). In British
Columbia, information about cost is available online from the BC
Cancer Agency, Screening Mammography Program 2017 Annual
Report, page 45 (http://www.bccancer.bc.ca/screening/Documents/
SMPAnnualReport2017_WEB.pdf).

Several attempts to obtain precise information about the cost in Ontario
failed as the Ontario Breast Screening Program reports costs for the
test, $20 million a year, but not for the costs of radiology staff and/or
infrastructure as these are contained within hospital and clinic budgets.

Acknowledgements

In 2014, I enrolled in the Master of Fine Arts in Creative Nonfiction program at the University of King's College in Halifax, wanting to write this book. I owe an enormous debt of gratitude to my writing mentors Kim Pittaway, Tim Falconer, and Harry Thurston, who patiently and skillfully guided my first draft. It was a privilege to work with such talented editors. I also thank my professors Donald Sedgwick and David Swick for their support and encouragement, as well as Stephen Kimber, one of the program's founders, for believing in my project and for his nurturing nudges. I'd also like to send a big shout-out to all of my MFA classmates, who continue to be generously encouraging and collegial. Without King's, I may never have dared to step into the writers' world.

I am delighted that my book found a home at Goose Lane Editions and thrilled that publisher Susanne Alexander trusted enough in what I was doing to take a chance with a controversial subject. To Karen Pinchin, former non-fiction acquisitions editor, thank you for championing the book. Many thanks to creative director Julie Scriver for a brilliant cover design that captures the essence of the narrative perfectly. I also thank production editor Alan Sheppard and publicist Jeff Arbeau for their professionalism and enthusiasm for the project. I owe special thanks to my hard-working and patient editors, Jill Ainsley, Holly Dickinson, and Jess Shulman for their wisdom, insights, and attention to detail. Thanks to everyone at team Goose Lane. I am proud to be one of your geese.

I will forever be grateful to my agents John Pearce and Chris Casuccio for taking on the project. From the beginning, they completely understood what the book is about and have been unwavering in their support. If I ever had a discouraging moment, they were there to paint the big picture and help me past the small stuff. I thank the Westwood Creative Artists group for being so welcoming.

I would like to mention some of my former colleagues at CBC News. Ioanna Roumeliotis, Melanie Glanz, Pauline Dakin, and Amina Zafar took on the assignment to report on the 2014 update of the Canadian National Breast Screening Study, under my supervision. As I worked with them to navigate the complexities of the story, I knew I had to write this book. I remember saying it out loud in the office. I owe them all for their inspiration. Another CBC colleague who deserves thanks is Arthur Schwartzel, video library coordinator, for his help in locating the videos referred to in the book.

There are many people to thank for the time they gave, not just for interviews but also for answering email queries and helping locate important articles in the medical literature. Thank you to Rita Well for lending personal Strax family material. I especially wish to thank Hazel Thornton for travelling two hours by train to meet me in London. I also want to thank Cornelia Baines and Anthony Miller for many hours of interviews and conversation and for access to their files and documents, some of which they both generously loaned to me.

Finally, I say thanks to my best friend and lifelong partner Jim Handman for standing by me, always, and for putting up with the many, many days I was so engrossin in the work I was barely approachable. Thank you, Jim, for your patience and support, for the research tips you constantly sent my way, for all the brilliant suggestions you made, and for never letting me lose sight of the goal.

Index

Women's Leadership Summit on
    Mammography 96
World Health Organization 24, 150
Wright, Charles 15, 68–73, 205

Y

Yaffe, Martin; early career 78–81;
    involvement in Canadian study
    82; criticisms of Canadian
    study 79, 81, 99–104, 108–11;
    involvement with Canadian
    Breast Cancer Foundation 226;
    3D mammography 79–81, 89
Young, Jennifer 230, 231

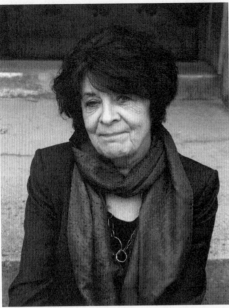

Renée Pellerin is a former television and radio producer with CBC. For many years, she was a documentary producer for *Marketplace*, specializing in investigative health stories. She was also a producer at the *Fifth Estate*, consultant to the CBC Newsworld program *Health Matters*, executive producer of a documentary unit at CBC Newsworld, and a producer at *Morningside* and *Sunday Morning*. Before she left CBC, she was the head of the Health Content Unit for CBC News, leading a team of health journalists in radio, TV, and online.

Pellerin has won several national and international awards for her work, including a Michener Citation of Merit for public service in journalism. She has also taught journalism at the National University of Rwanda in Butare and at Ryerson University in Toronto, and has held the visiting chair in journalism at the University of Regina. She holds degrees from the University of Saskatchewan and University of King's College in Halifax. She now lives in Niagara-on-the-Lake.